SECRETS OF
AYURVEDA

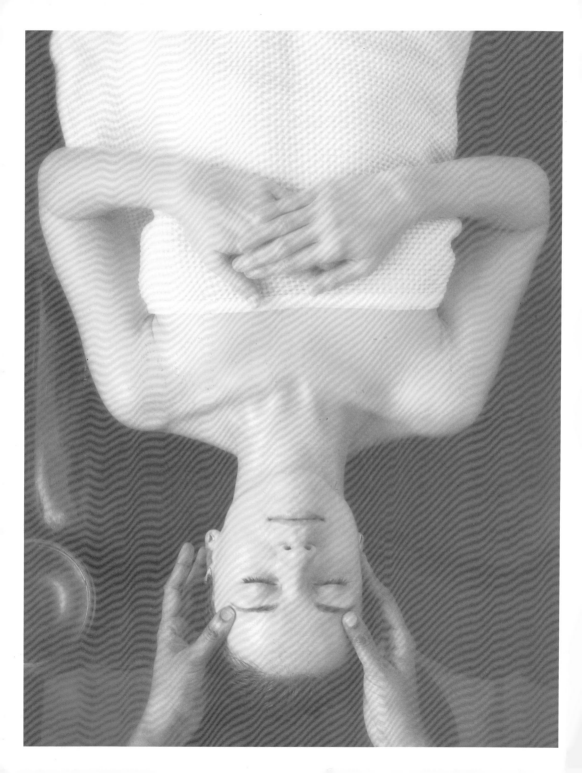

SECRETS OF
AYURVEDA

GOPI WARRIER, DR HARISH VERMA
& KAREN SULLIVAN

IVY PRESS

This edition published in the UK and North America in 2017 by
Ivy Press
An imprint of The Quarto Group
The Old Brewery, 6 Blundell Street
London N7 9BH, United Kingdom
T (0)20 7700 6700 F (0)20 7700 8066
www.QuartoKnows.com

First published in 2001

British Library Cataloguing-in-Publication Data
A catalogue record for this book is available from the British Library

ISBN: 978-1-78240-492-7

This book was conceived, designed and produced by
Ivy Press
58 West Street, Brighton BN1 2RA, United Kingdom

Art Director: Peter Bridgewater
Publisher: Sophie Collins
Editorial Director: Steve Luck
Designers: Siân Keogh, Sandra Marques and Ginny Zeal
Editors: Kim Davies and Mary Devine
Picture Researcher: Mary Devine
Photography: David Jordan and Guy Ryecart
Photography organization: Kim Davies and Siân Keogh
Illustrations: Axis Design Editions Limited, Michael Courtney, Catherine
McIntyre, Andrew Kulman, Stephen Raw and Sarah Young
Three-dimensional models: Mark Jamieson
Assistant Editor: Jenny Campbell

Printed in China

10 9 8 7 6 5 4 3 2 1

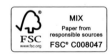

Note from the publisher
Information given in this book is not intended to be taken as a replacement
for medical advice. Any person with a condition requiring medical attention
should consult a qualified medical practitioner or therapist.

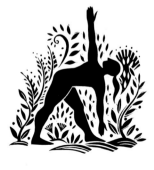

Cover image: Shutterstock/Nataliia Kucherenko

How to Use This Book   6

Introduction   8

Chapter 1: **Ayurveda: The Science of Life**   **10**

Chapter 2: **The Ayurvedic Approach**   **66**

Chapter 3: **Diet & Lifestyle**   **150**

Chapter 4: **Practitioner-led or Self-help?**   **190**

Glossary   216

Further Reading   217

Useful Addresses   218

Index   220

Acknowledgments   224

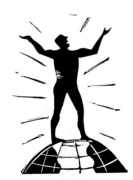
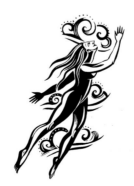
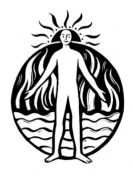

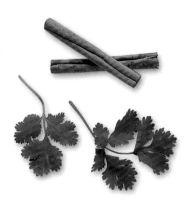

A natural system
*Ayurveda uses herbs, diet,
massage, and other therapies,
to enhance well-being.*

HOW TO USE THIS BOOK

Ayurveda is a complete medical system that has been used for thousands of years. This book explains the principles behind it clearly and simply and is suitable for complete beginners. To make it easy to use, this fully illustrated guide has been divided into four chapters. The first takes you through the fascinating history of Ayurveda and helps you to pinpoint your Ayurvedic constitution. The therapies and routines of Ayurveda are fully expanded in the second and third chapters, with a complete section devoted to diet. Finally, it explains when you need to see a practitioner and how to use Ayurveda at home.

Important Notice

Ayurvedic medicine is a holistic approach to health. The claims in this book have been sincerely made, but neither the publisher nor the authors can be held responsible for any claim or belief described. If you have a medical or psychiatric condition, you are advised to consult your doctor before seeing an Ayurvedic practitioner. The suggestions in this book are not intended as substitutes for medical or psychiatric treatment.

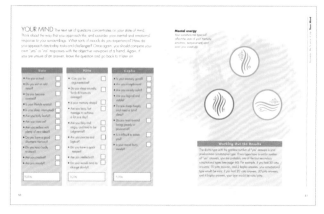

Diagnosis
*Simple questionnaires will help you
to work out your constitutional type.*

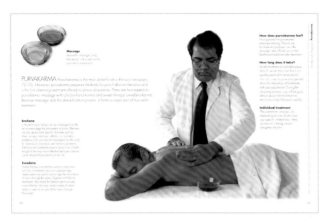

Therapies

These pages explain how an Ayurvedic doctor can help you.

Theories

These pages explain the theory behind Ayurvedic practice.

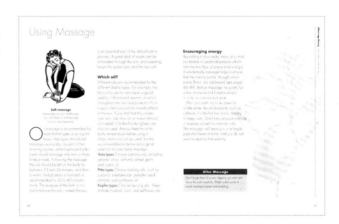

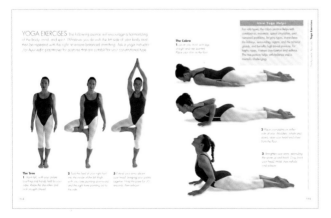

Self-help

Many of the pages offer practical ideas that you can use at home.

What Is Ayurveda?

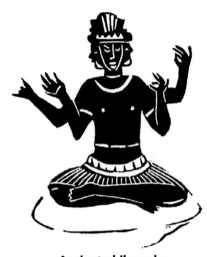

Ancient philosophy
Ayurveda calls upon the philosophy, wisdom, religion, and mythology of India.

Ayurveda is the system of healing practiced in India, Nepal, and Sri Lanka. Like Traditional Chinese Medicine (TCM), Ayurveda is a complete system, with a variety of components aimed at improving emotional, physical, and mental health. Thousands of years old, the discipline was established before the birth of the Buddha, and some biblical stories reflect the wisdom of Ayurvedic teachings.

The practice of Ayurveda is divided into many different branches, in order to encompass all aspects of health and healing. Medicine is only one spoke on the Ayurvedic wheel, and to benefit fully from Ayurveda, it is helpful to consider the other elements, including astrology, meditation, yoga, massage, sound and music therapy, breathing exercises, and much, much more.

The approach is vastly different from conventional Western medicine in some ways. It can be considered as a program for living, which addresses every part of human life and puts it into the context of our environment.

That is not to say that adopting every element of Ayurveda is essential for health and well-being, but by following a simple Ayurvedic approach, we can develop ways to remain balanced in times of increasing stress, pressure, and worry. Most importantly, we can adopt a lifestyle that works to create harmony, preventing illness and encouraging us to heal much more quickly when we do become ill.

Ayurvedic history

Ayurveda is a combination of science and philosophy, which details the many physical, mental, emotional, and spiritual aspects necessary for health. Ayurveda is said to have been handed down divinely by Lord Brahma, the creator of the universe according to Hindu mythology, through the divine Hindu books called *Vedas*.

The Vedas are: the *Rig Veda* (the oldest), the *Yajus Veda* and the *Sama Veda* (the backbone of Indian philosophy and religion dating from 3000 BCE), and the *Atharava*, the main source for Ayurveda, dating from 1200 BCE.

Medicinal knowledge is said to have been revealed by the god Indra to the sage Atreya, leading to the Charaka tradition of medicine. Ayurvedic books were written from 600 BCE to 1000 CE by Charaka, Sushruta, and Vaghbhatta.

Divine Revelation

Surgery is said to have been revealed to the king Devodas, and this led to the Sushruta tradition of Ayurvedic surgery.

AYURVEDA:
THE SCIENCE OF LIFE

Ayurveda literally means "the science of life." It is a Sanskrit word, derived from two roots: *ayus* and *vid*, meaning "life" and "knowledge." *Ayus* are daily life cycles that represent the body, the senses, the mind, and the soul. *Veda* is a knowledge of our world and how everything within it works. The great *rishis* (seers or wise men) of ancient India established a system of belief called Vedic philosophy that offered new insight into the concepts of sickness and health. From there, they organized the sophisticated science of living known as Ayurveda, which takes into consideration the physical, mental, emotional, and spiritual elements of life necessary for health and well-being. For this reason, Ayurveda is holistic, meaning that it addresses health on every level.

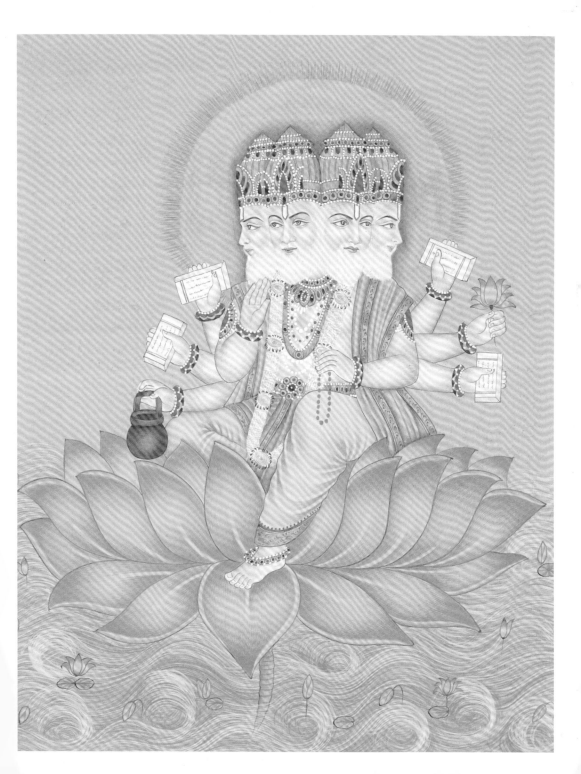

Understanding Ayurveda

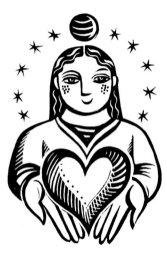

A natural balance
Restoring balance to the mind, body, and soul is the aim of Ayurveda.

The ancient system of Ayurveda teaches that all illnesses affect both the body and the mind, and never treats either in isolation from the other. Ayurvedic medicine can be simple and straightforward, such as using a herbal remedy for a sore throat or headache, or more profound, for example, taking into consideration our health in previous lives as a basis for gaining or preserving good health in this one.

The Western perspective

In the West, we take the view that people are fundamentally the same, and we treat "conditions" rather than the individual who is suffering. Ayurveda addresses the uniqueness of each patient, taking into consideration the state of the mind and spirit as well as physical health. Diagnosis is based on the patient's constitution.

A modern approach

Although Ayurveda is over 3,000 years old, it has changed dramatically with the times, as lifestyle, diet, and the demands placed on the body have altered. In fact, many modern conditions, such as irritable bowel syndrome and Chronic Fatigue Syndrome have been successfully treated by Ayurveda when conventional medicine has failed. Far from being a system of living based on an out-of-date mythology, Ayurveda is a relevant, dynamic, advanced health system which has been proved to be scientifically accurate.

Toward good health

In Vedic philosophy, our lives become meaningful when we strive to fulfill our potential, but this cannot be achieved without basic good health. Ayurvedic theory is based on the constitution of the individual, which dictates his or her susceptibility to certain illnesses.

Ayurveda takes into account the influence of psychosomatic factors in most diseases as well as any imbalance in the individual's basic constitution. Ayurveda concentrates on preserving well-being, and on improving our spiritual, intellectual, and physical ability to heal ourselves. Treatment is aimed at restoring balance of the basic constitutional factors, or doshas (see pages 30–31).

Divine Medicine

In India there is a saying that wealth earned from medical practice is contaminated since it is gained from the suffering of others. Ayurveda is said to have been handed down divinely and should therefore be practiced with compassion and nobility, not greed or egotism.

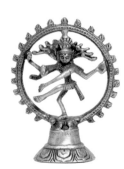

Religious roots
Ayurveda emphasizes the spiritual side of life and has its origins in Hinduism.

A HISTORY OF AYURVEDA Ayurveda has a rich and varied history, much of which is intertwined with Indian mythology. Although Ayurveda is believed to be eternal and universal, belonging to no particular country, religion, or civilization, its roots are in the East—in particular, in the *Charaka Samhita*. This remarkable document of internal medicine, which was written more than 2,000 years before the microscope was invented, explains how the body is made up of cells and lists 20 different microscopic organisms which may cause disease.

Origins

Ancient Ayurvedic wisdom tells us that thousands of years ago, the rishis (wise men) were disheartened by the suffering of humanity. They realized that ill health and decreasing lifespans allowed people little time to attend to their spirituality. Fifty-two rishis traveled to the foot of the Himalayas to learn how to cleanse the world of illness.

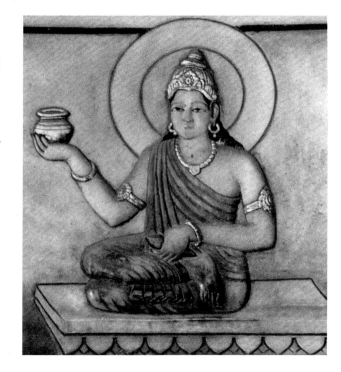

Pathway to health
In Ayurveda, spirituality is seen as the cornerstone of well-being in this world and thereafter.

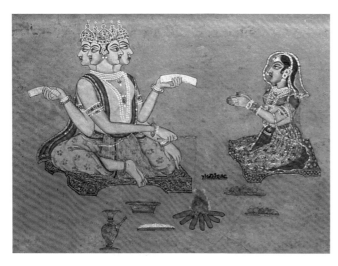

Brahma's gift
*The Vedas, sacred texts that form
the basis for Ayurvedic knowledge,
were revealed by Lord Brahma,
the Hindu creator of the universe.*

The birth of Ayurveda
The 52 rishis meditated together and, through this
spiritual practice, acquired the knowledge that
was then written down as Ayurveda. The principal
text, known as the *Charaka Samhita*, is considered
sacred. Three aspects of the knowledge were
passed on to the rishis—etiology (the science of
the cause of disease), symptomatology (the study
and interpretation of symptoms), and medication.

Demonic disease
Until the advent of Ayurveda, disease was
explained in terms of possession by various
demonic disease entities. A body afflicted by
disease caused the spirit to be weighed down
by worldly concerns, preventing enlightenment
and physical and mental health.

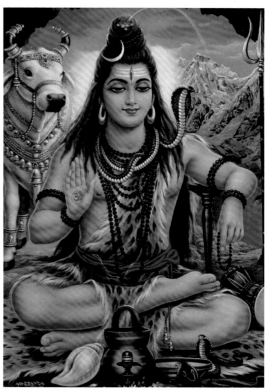

Lord of healing
*Shiva is one of the Hindu gods
for healing. He is worshipped
for the cure of diseases.*

The Origins of Ayurveda

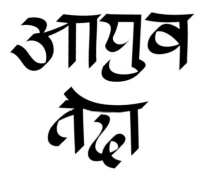

Ayus & vid
The sanskrit ayus, *meaning
"life," and* vid, *"science," are the
root words for Ayurveda,
"the science of life."*

S ome experts believe that the earliest
Ayurvedic teachings were those
contained in the sacred writings of
Hinduism, the Vedas, although this cannot
be proven. There are four Vedas in all, and
Atharva Veda, part of the fourth, contains
one of the earliest detailed accounts of the
system of Ayurveda. From this and other
texts (see page 15), Ayurvedic medicine
was developed. Through the centuries
that have followed, the system has been
adapted in order to help people best at
different points in time.

Spreading the word
Asoka, who was the emperor of
India from about 272 to 231 BCE,
was responsible for establishing many
Ayurvedic hospitals. He also sent
disciples to the Far and Middle East,
and the philosophy of Ayurveda
eventually spread from India into the
healing practices of China, Arabia,
Persia, and Greece.

We now know that Ayurvedic
practitioners reached ancient Athens
and that traditional Greek medicine
was based on an idea of different bodily
humors, or constitutions, which can be
related to the principle of the three doshas
in Ayurveda—*vata, kapha,* and *pitta*
(see pages 30–31). Greek medicine was
extremely influential in the development
of traditional Western medicine.

Ayurvedic influences on Chinese
medicine are obvious: both disciplines
use energy points, pulse diagnosis, and
herbal remedies. The five elements used
in Chinese medicine may have their
root in Ayurvedic *panchamahabhutas*
(see pages 54–55).

The 20th century

Ayurveda was the principal system of medicine practiced in India until the beginning of the 20th century, when colonial rule began to favor Western medical techniques and labeled Ayurveda "out of date." Many wealthy families encouraged their children to study Western medicine, and Ayurveda all but died out.

However, in 1980, the National Congress of India decreed that Ayurveda should enjoy equal status with Western medicine. Today, Ayurveda is a thriving science, and more than 500 new Ayurvedic companies and hospitals have been established in India during the last ten years. Orthodox doctors and Ayurvedic physicians are now to be found working together.

A Transcendental Yogi

Ayurveda was brought to the West in the 1960s by Maharishi Mahesh Yogi, the Indian guru of Transcendental Meditation. He lectured in the U.S. and Germany and numbered the Beatles among his followers.

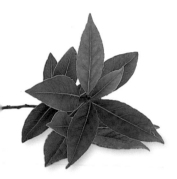

A herbal legacy
Ayurvedic medicines are based on natural ingredients and prepared from herbs.

THE EIGHT BRANCHES
The practice of Ayurvedic medicine includes eight branches. Practitioners—known as *vaidyas*—are well trained in the principles of nutrition, psychology, herbalism, climatology, and, in most cases, gem therapy and astrology as well.

A holistic approach
The aim of Ayurveda is not only healing the sick, but prevention of illness and the preservation of life. The Ayurvedic theory of creation discusses several factors which are interlinked, including:
• the body;
• the mind;
• the soul (consciousness);
• the panchamahabhutas (five elements).
These four factors are complementary to each other, and are equally important in every individual.

Tree of life
Ayurveda includes all branches of medicine from pediatrics to older people; from herbal medicine to general and plastic surgery.

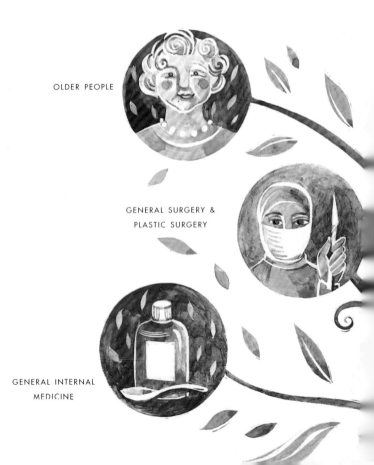

OLDER PEOPLE

GENERAL SURGERY & PLASTIC SURGERY

GENERAL INTERNAL MEDICINE

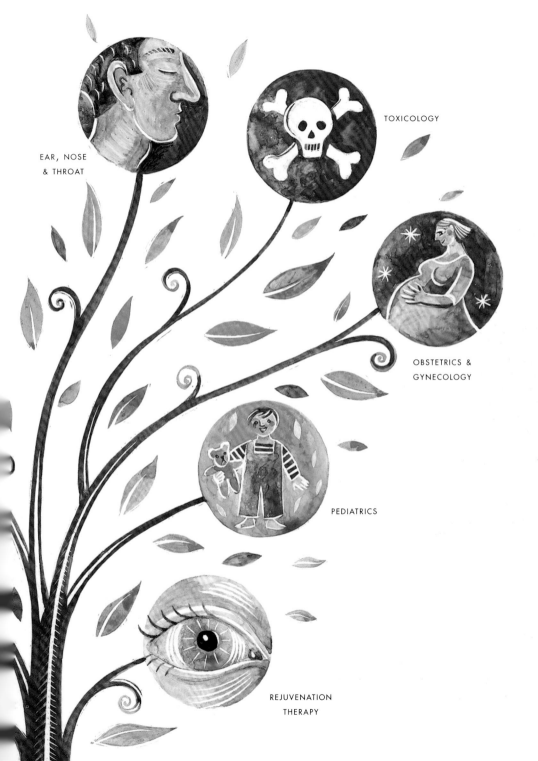

EAR, NOSE
& THROAT

TOXICOLOGY

OBSTETRICS &
GYNECOLOGY

PEDIATRICS

REJUVENATION
THERAPY

The Law of Karma

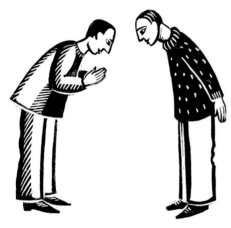

Harmonious living
*Ayurveda embraces the idea
that the path to harmony is
through moral living.*

Karma is the Hindu belief of reciprocity. In other words, it is a belief that every action has an equal and opposite reaction. Karma is an integral part of all Eastern religions, including Buddhism and Jainism, as well as Hinduism, and appears in all the different schools of Hindu philosophy.

The concept of karma also forms the foundation of the theory of reincarnation. Reincarnation is the belief that all human and animal life goes through the cycles of birth and rebirth until such time as they attain a state of "perfection." At this point, they are ready for deliverance or liberation from the cycle of repeated births in this world, whose nature is essentially that of suffering. This liberation, called *moksha*, is the ultimate goal of all beings incarnated in this world.

According to Ayurveda, disease is the product of karma. No other theory can adequately explain the suffering of noble individuals and children in this world. This theory does not suggest the idea of a cruel god but of a just and balanced universal being and consciousness, within which all positive and negative forces are automatically adjusted to ensure the harmonious existence of the whole.

The forms of karma

In Hinduism, there are three types of karma for individuals:

• *Prarabdha karma* is karma that you are born with, and it relates to the karma of your past life. In other words, if you were a cruel husband in a previous life, it will have an impact upon your marriage in this or a future life. You may even end up with a cruel wife in another lifetime.

- *Sanchita karma* relates to karma that you have accumulated during your current lifetime through your actions and your thoughts.
- *Agama karma* is the karma that you can create by future action in this life, or in future lives.

According to Ayurveda, ailments caused by accumulated negative karma cannot be cured by medical treatment alone. Indian astrology (see pages 142–45) can be used to understand the nature of your individual karma, the karmic causes of diseases, and, therefore, to what extent you will be able to cure your illnesses through medical treatment.

Clearing the Karma

There is a clear statement in *Charaka Samhita*, the sacred Ayurvedic text, which says that "all diseases can only be fully cured when the karma that has caused it is fully expiated."

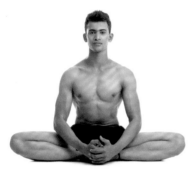

Hidden way
Ayurveda holds the belief that regular spiritual exercise, such as meditation, can benefit health.

CAUSE & EFFECT
The meaning of karma has shifted through the centuries but has always revolved around the notion of action, especially religious action. The concept has come to refer to acts, good or bad, that result in positive or negative outcomes. Major illnesses, prolonged ailments, infertility, acute and disfiguring skin diseases, and mental illnesses can be, according to Ayurveda, the outcomes of bad karma.

Serious ailments
The remedies for diseases that are caused by karma are prayer and spiritual action, devotional practices, and the use of mantras. Most Ayurvedic practitioners will vouch that for serious ailments these remedies are at least partially, if not fully, effective in healing disease.

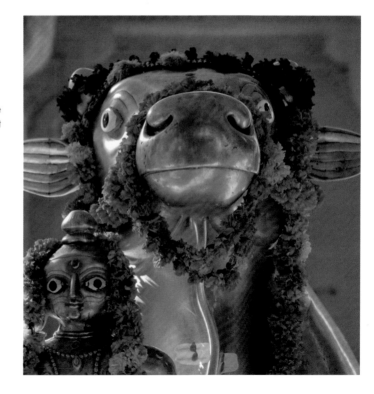

Releasing karma
Spiritual devotion takes many forms, and can be used to release negative karma.

The Effect of Karma

Bodily events
The quality of our health may be dependent on our accumulated past karma.

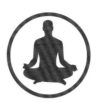

Perceptions
Our understanding of the world governs the way we relate to it.

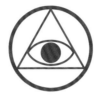

Feelings
Negative emotions can encourage bad karma.

Disposition
Our temperament may be the result of actions in previous lives.

Consciousness
According to karmic law, our soul or spirit continues after physical death.

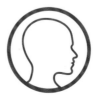

The Concept of Balance

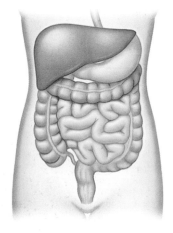

A healthy system

A vital part of remaining healthy is to ensure good elimination of waste products from the body.

In the practice of Ayurveda, health is more than just an absence of disease. It involves a harmonious interaction between the emotions, intellect, body, actions, behavior, and the environment in which we live. All of these elements are equally important. Balance is health in Ayurvedic philosophy.

When we reach a state of balance, we achieve an inner harmony that brings with it a profound contentment and sense of well-being. On a physical level, we are considered to be healthy when all of our various functions (including our digestion, metabolism, elimination, and tissues) are in balance.

And just as important to physical health are the states of our mind, soul, and senses, which should be peaceful, content, and happy.

Causes of imbalance

Apart from the factors mentioned on pages 22–23, there are a number of reasons why we lose our equilibrium. When we work against our nature over a prolonged period of time, perhaps by eating badly, living inappropriately, or experiencing periods of stress and negative emotions, our health will break down and we will become sick. This is because the doshas (see pages 30–31) have become unbalanced for one or more of these reasons.

Detoxification

When our vital energies are unbalanced over a long period of time, illness often results. The main damage caused by a state of imbalance is a build-up of *ama* (see page 65), which are toxins and waste products. One of the first treatments that Ayurvedic medicine offers is a five-fold detoxification procedure called *panchakarma*, which aims to rid the body of ama in order to restore the balance between the three doshas.

True Health

In the *Charaka Samhita*, Ayurveda's principal text, health is said to exist when all of the following conditions are present:

- All three doshas (*vata*, *pitta*, and *kapha*) are perfectly balanced

- The five senses are functioning naturally

- The body, mind, and spirit are in harmony

- All the tissues of the body (*dhaatus*) are functioning properly

- The three *malas* (the waste products, urine, feces, and sweat) are produced and naturally eliminated

- The channels of the body (the equivalent of meridians, known as *srotas*) are unblocked and flowing with energy

- The digestive fire or *agni* (metabolism in Western terms) is healthy and the appetite is working normally.

HEALTH & SICKNESS

The purpose of Ayurvedic medicine is to ensure that we can avoid serious illness by understanding how we become sick and by avoiding unhealthy practices. When illness does strike, there is a wide range of treatments that help the body to heal itself. The first objective of Ayurvedic therapy is to restore any imbalance between the vital life energies. The next stage is designed to establish a long-term stability (balance) between the energies and to produce a state of optimum health and well-being.

Is the theory important?

Much Ayurvedic theory is complicated and difficult to understand from a Western perspective. However, it is important to understand why exercises are performed, why routines must be undertaken, how and when we should eat and sleep, and all of the other aspects of the therapy. It is believed that in order to attain optimum health and well-being, we need to increase our awareness and respect for the spirit.

Quiet time

Sitting quietly for half an hour every day helps to increase awareness of the spiritual self.

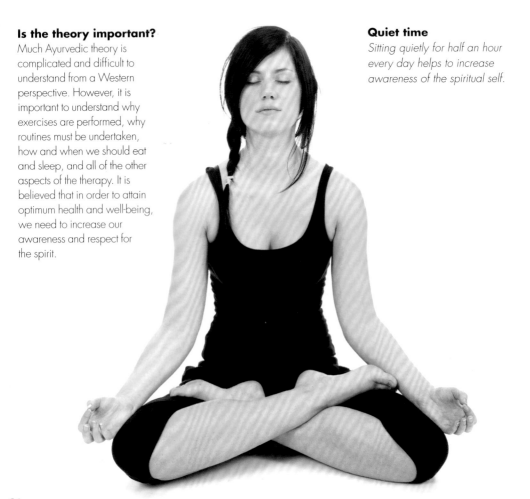

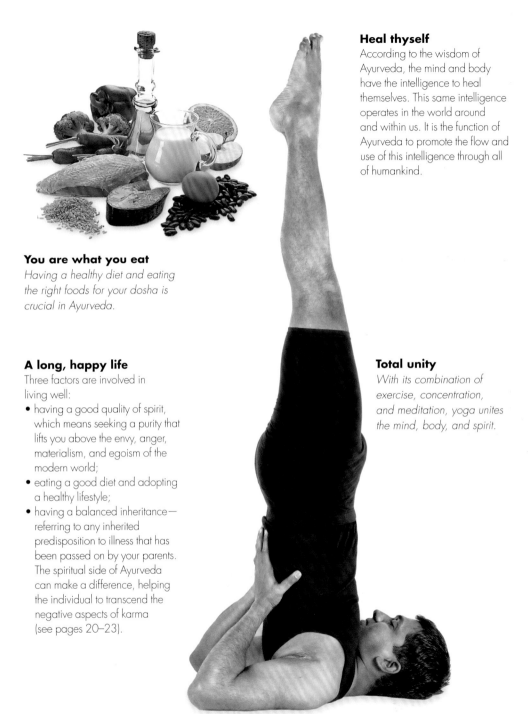

Heal thyself

According to the wisdom of Ayurveda, the mind and body have the intelligence to heal themselves. This same intelligence operates in the world around and within us. It is the function of Ayurveda to promote the flow and use of this intelligence through all of humankind.

You are what you eat

Having a healthy diet and eating the right foods for your dosha is crucial in Ayurveda.

A long, happy life

Three factors are involved in living well:

- having a good quality of spirit, which means seeking a purity that lifts you above the envy, anger, materialism, and egoism of the modern world;
- eating a good diet and adopting a healthy lifestyle;
- having a balanced inheritance— referring to any inherited predisposition to illness that has been passed on by your parents. The spiritual side of Ayurveda can make a difference, helping the individual to transcend the negative aspects of karma (see pages 20–23).

Total unity

With its combination of exercise, concentration, and meditation, yoga unites the mind, body, and spirit.

27

The Cause of Disease

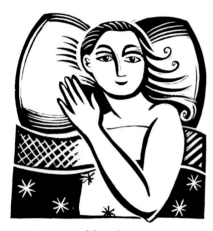

Healthy sleep
*Getting enough sleep
is one factor that can help
to ensure good health.*

In Ayurveda, many factors are believed to cause disease, and some may seem unusual to Western readers. For example, it is believed that evil spirits can be at the root of some problems. Although this may not be a popular Western view, research into multiple-personality disorders has, in some instances, given this theory credence. Other causes include poisons, toxins, fire, pollution, accidents, planetary activity, acts of God, and karmic influences.

Unhealthy behavior

The true cause of disease in Ayurvedic terms is imbalance. Three main factors can lead to imbalance.

• Misuse of the mind and body (*prajnaparadha*), including all thoughts or actions that breach the natural order of human life and impair the intellect, emotions, and memory. Causes in this category could include neglecting your body and health, overusing alcohol, suppressing natural physical urges, such as coughing, yawning, sneezing, defecating, or urinating, acting selfishly, or befriending unsuitable (greedy, hate-filled, or angry) people.

• Unhealthy association of the sense organs with sense objects (*asatmyendriyartha samyoga*). This means the under- or over-stimulation of the five sense organs. Listening to loud, piercing noises, including some music, living in unhygienic circumstances, sniffing intoxicating substances, or overdoing some body therapies, including massage, are all examples of unhealthy associations.

• Influences of time and the season (see pages 132–33). According to Ayurveda, a series of routines form the foundation of life. Some are undertaken on a daily basis, some yearly, and others at different points in life. Furthermore, our lives are believed to be set in cycles. All these cycles are important and must be adhered to in order to attain good health. For example, not getting enough sleep or exposing yourself to excessive cold in winter or heat in summer are considered detrimental. In Ayurveda, many diseases are seasonal, and treatment varies from one time of year to another. Each of the three doshas increases during its season; it is important for those with a predominant dosha to pay special attention during its season to keep their dosha balanced.

Cause of Disease

The main cause of disease is an imbalance of the doshas, which are the three bodily energies that influence all living matter. The imbalance can be sudden or slow to appear.

THE THREE DOSHAS

Central to the philosophy of Ayurveda is the belief that we are composed of three vital energies, known as the doshas. Each of us is born with an individual constitution. Our constitution is determined by the state of our parents' doshas at the time of conception and other factors. Each of us is born in the *prakruthi* state, which means that we are born with levels of the three doshas that are right for us. The best defense against illness is a strong constitution. If our doshas become imbalanced, through bad habits, food, or overwork, for example, we become susceptible to illness. Ayurveda helps to prevent the development of disease by working with the constitution of the individual, aiming to restore it to its prakruthi state.

What are the doshas?

Each of us has a unique constitution, which is determined by the balance of vital energies in the body—the three doshas, or tridosha. The three doshas are known by their Sanskrit names of *vata*, *pitta*, and *kapha*. Everyone's constitution is governed by all three doshas in varying degrees, but most of us are also governed by one or possibly two dominant doshas.

A healthy constitution

The best defense against illness is a good constitution. If our bodies are functioning well, disease is unlikely, but when the constitution is weakened we become susceptible to illness. Ayurveda aims to prevent disease, working with the individual's constitution.

Influence of the doshas

Our dosha determines our constitution, preferences, personality traits, sleeping patterns, and even the foods we should eat. As we go through life, environment, diet, stress, trauma, and injury cause the doshas to become unbalanced, a condition known as the *vikruthi* state. When the imbalance is excessively high or low it can lead to ill health.

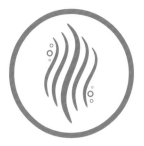

Vata
Vata types are connected to the elements of ether and air.

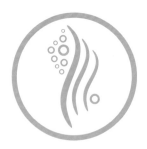

Pitta
Pitta types are connected to the elements of fire and water.

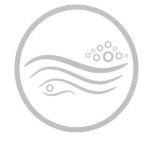

Kapha
Kapha types are connected to the elements of water and earth.

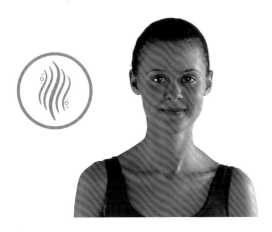

Vata type
Vatas are often thin, with dry skin, long, angular faces, small eyes, irregular teeth, and narrow lips.

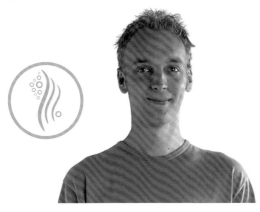

Pitta type
Pittas are often fair and freckled, with heart-shaped faces, neat noses, and pale eyes. Their teeth may be yellowish.

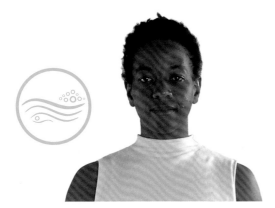

Kapha type
Kaphas may be oily-skinned, with thick wavy hair, blue or brown eyes, and solid builds.

Characteristics of the Three Vital Forces

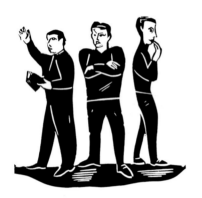

One of a kind

Although every one of us is unique, we all conform to one of the three dosha types or a combination of them.

The concept of the tridoshas is unique to Ayurvedic philosophy, according to which there are three vital forces, vata, pitta, and kapha. These govern the entire physical and mental functions in the living being. When these vital forces are in balance, they provide good health and longevity for the human being, and when they are imbalanced, they are responsible for diseases and ill health.

Three types of dosha

Each dosha type has different characteristics. Vata types tend to be thin and restless with poor teeth, a tendency to bite their nails, and erratic sleep patterns. Pitta types tend to be of medium frame and height. They are most likely to have a reddish or yellowish complexion and often have green, gray, or brown eyes. They will be natural leaders but will have a tendency towards jealousy and anger and may be judgmental.

Kapha types have strong, well-proportioned bodies, with a tendency toward excess weight. They usually have a strong sexual desire and a regular, steady appetite. They are intelligent and speak clearly and have strong immune systems.

Biological processes

The doshas govern all of the biological processes, and their energies govern our physical and psychological make-up. This means that the predominant force within each of us defines the following:

- our physical appearance;
- the internal functioning of our organs;
- our intellectual capacity;
- our temperament.

Most people conform to a type that is a mixture of two doshas, with one more dominant than the other. The prevailing dosha determines not only the above factors but our predisposition to particular conditions or disorders.

Each of the three doshas takes five forms within the body, according to its function and the site of activity. For example, the five types of vata in the body are *prana* (found in the head), *udana* (chest), *vyana* (heart), *apana* (pelvis), and *samana* (stomach).

Age & the Doshas

From childhood to teens we are influenced by kapha, from 20 to 50 the influence is pitta, and from 60 onward, the influence is vata.

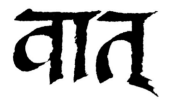

Vata

The Sanskrit word vata *means "to move," and vata people have powerful, mobile natures.*

VATA *Vata* is a Sanskrit word meaning "to move," or "to enthuse." Vata forms the most important constituent of the tridosha framework and is responsible for the movements of the body (both physical and mental). Vata upholds the supportive structure and tissue and governs circulation throughout the body. The cosmic link of vata is wind, and its main principle is change. Its elements are ether and air (see below), and it influences activity and movement. Therefore, the vata type will be susceptible to excess wind and air, and will be changeable, with an active lifestyle and/or personality.

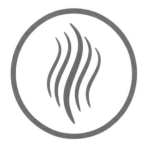

Air

Air is one of the eternal substances that combine with the soul to create a being.

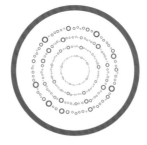

Ether

Ether, or space, corresponds to the spaces in the body, such as the mouth and nostrils.

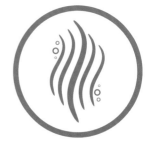

Air/ether

Vata's elements are ether and air, the cosmic link is wind, and its principle is change.

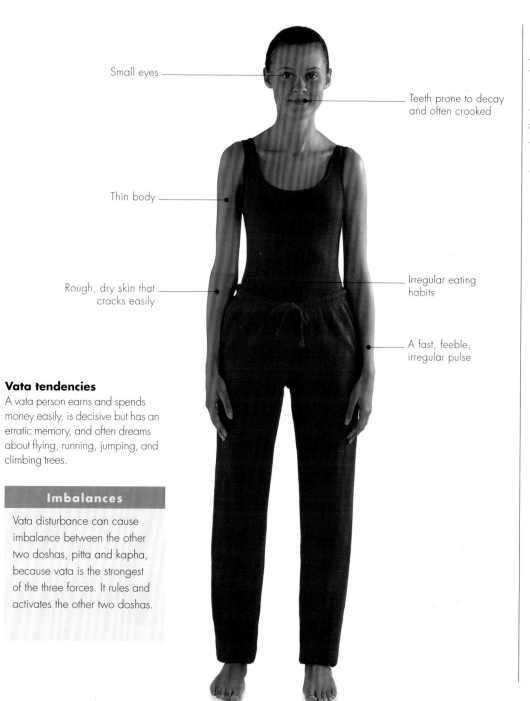

Small eyes

Teeth prone to decay and often crooked

Thin body

Rough, dry skin that cracks easily

Irregular eating habits

A fast, feeble, irregular pulse

Vata tendencies

A vata person earns and spends money easily, is decisive but has an erratic memory, and often dreams about flying, running, jumping, and climbing trees.

Imbalances

Vata disturbance can cause imbalance between the other two doshas, pitta and kapha, because vata is the strongest of the three forces. It rules and activates the other two doshas.

Vata Imbalances

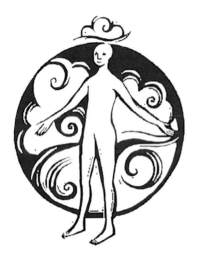

The center of the storm

A vata imbalance can be caused by fast living and is exacerbated by the wind.

What causes imbalance?

The Western lifestyle is the main culprit, and vata is naturally drawn to exciting experiences and fast living. Stress, too much activity, an inability to relax, over-indulgence in food, tobacco, and alcohol, overwork, and too much physical or emotional strain can all cause an imbalance when allowed to continue for long periods of time. Even adventure vacations—which naturally appeal to vatas—with plenty of challenging activities can aggravate vata. For this reason it is often recommended that vata types take vacations in a warm, relaxing environment, where there are not too many distractions. Other causes of disturbance in vata include skipping meals, inadequate sleep, cold, windy weather, and eating too much raw, cold, or dry food.

Vata relates to stress and the nervous system and also to depletion, and our Western lifestyles can play havoc with these. Vata people can easily suffer from anxiety, fear, grief, or agitation, largely because they take on life at full steam. If you find you are predominantly vata (see page 48–51), try to take time out to recharge your batteries on a regular basis. Slow down the pace of life and spend time on gentle pursuits.

Signs of balanced vata

When vata is in balance with the other doshas, the vata person will be enthusiastic, focused, and positive. The stereotypical vata type has the ability to act quickly, to adapt to new situations easily, and to be alert and creative. When vata is balanced, the vata type sleeps well, has efficient elimination from both bladder and bowel, and has a very strong immune system.

Signs of Imbalance

All of the following symptoms, or combinations of symptoms, can be telltale signs that vata is in a state of imbalance.

- Rough skin
- Brittle, rough fingernails
- Dry tongue
- Grayish-brown complexion
- Constipation
- Hacking cough
- Dry eyes or lips
- Depression or a loss of energy and joy in life
- Respiratory disorders
- Insomnia or interrupted sleep
- Nonspecific fatigue
- Anxiety, worry, and confusion
- Dizziness
- High blood pressure
- Muscle tensions
- Nervous pain
- Trembling or shivering
- Cramps
- Weight loss
- "Nervous" stomach upsets

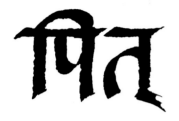

Pitta

The Sanskrit word pitta *means "heating" or "burning," and can denote a fiery temperament.*

PITTA *Pitta* is a Sanskrit word meaning "to heat" or "to burn." It is responsible for all biochemical activities, including the production of heat, and is made up of fire and water elements. Pitta's cosmic link is the sun, and its main principle is conversion. It influences metabolism or transformation. The pitta type will have a tendency toward "excess fire," and will be able to transform or change things easily. The fire in the pitta nature creates a tendency toward anger, sudden outbreaks of bad temper, and being judgmental. Pittas are often considered overly competitive.

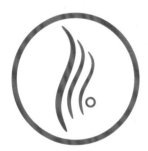

Fire

Pitta types are often excessively fiery, which is caused by the cosmic link to the sun.

Water

Water represents conversion, and pitta types are often able to make changes easily.

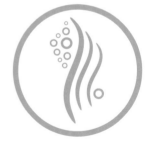

Fire/water

Pitta is made up of fire and water, and two of its natural qualities are fluidity and heat.

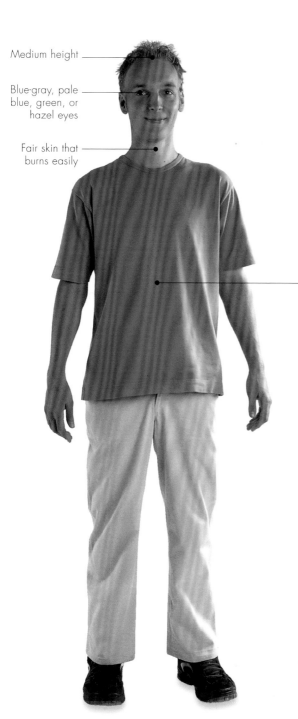

Medium height

Blue-gray, pale blue, green, or hazel eyes

Fair skin that burns easily

Often hungry, with large appetite

Pitta tendencies

In general pittas are decisive, open to new ideas, and skilled in using words, although they dislike overwork. The pitta pulse is known as "the frog" because it jumps around; the resting pulse is about 70–80 bpm and tends to be erratic.

Pitta Types

The five types of pitta are:

- *Paachaku* (found in the stomach). This is the most important pitta energy. It helps the others function and affects the digestive juices;

- *Ranjana* (in the spleen, stomach, and liver). The liver ranjana is most important, because of the liver's vital role in detoxification;

- Saadhaka (in the heart) governs intelligence, intellect, memory, creativity, self-esteem, and romance;

- *Aalochaka* (in the pupils) influences the ability to see external objects;

- *Bhraajaka* (in the skin) regulates body temperature, sweating, and oil secretion.

Pitta Imbalances

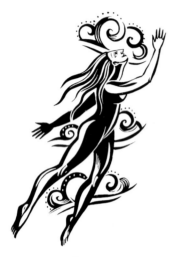

High energy
*Pitta types have a burning desire
that can often manifest itself as
over-ambition.*

P itta people are normally healthy and
strong, with good immunity. Although
they are not as driven as the vata type,
pitta types often have to learn to relax
because their high energy levels keep
them going when others around them
have flagged. Because pitta is associated
with the main element of fire, you can
expect a fiery personality from time to
time, sometimes resulting in jealousy,
competitiveness, and over-ambition.

What causes imbalance?

Like vata types, the pitta type can become
unbalanced by prolonged stress and an
erratic lifestyle. It is important, therefore,
to ensure that you get plenty of sleep, do
not miss meals, and take time to express
emotion that may bubble up. Other causes
of imbalance include excess heat or
sunlight, and salty, greasy, or spicy foods,
leading to digestive problems. Pitta is
aggravated when you watch television, use
a computer, or walk while you are eating.

Signs of balanced pitta

When this fiery element is well balanced
in a pitta type, there will be high energy
levels, with an accompanying feeling of
contentment, inner peace, harmony, and
well-being. Appetite will be strong and
digestion good. Pitta musculature will be
graceful, skin will be soft, the hormones
will be balanced (reducing the likelihood
of hormonal problems, such as PMS),
and the liver will effectively reduce toxin
levels in the body. Most importantly,
however, the pitta type will experience
heightened intellectual abilities, creativity,
and success. Pittas are advised to drink

plenty of water and to maintain a cool environment where possible. In fact, pittas are advised to live near water.

Signs of Imbalance

All of the following symptoms, or combinations of symptoms, can be telltale signs that pitta is in a state of imbalance.

- Profuse sweating and hot flashes
- Bad breath
- Sleep problems
- Poor digestion
- Weak liver
- Hormone deficiencies
- Heartburn
- Eczema
- Excessive hunger
- Yellowish complexion and blotchy skin
- Inflammatory conditions
- Irritable bowel syndrome

Fiery Temperament

Pitta emotions are fiery—jealousy, hatred, rage, and anger are common. They can, however, subside as quickly as they flare up.

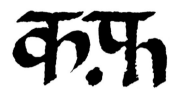

Kapha
The Sanskrit word kapha *means "embracing," and kapha types tend to be forgiving and loving.*

KAPHA
Kapha is a Sanskrit word meaning "to embrace" or "to keep together." Kapha is a source of both strength and resistance and is responsible for the construction of the living body. Kapha is made up of the water and earth elements. Because of its composition (earth is stabilizing), kapha is steadier than the other two doshas. The cosmic link is the moon and the main principle is inertia, which means that kapha types must have stimulation in order to avoid boredom. The kapha type is usually good at holding things together and does not like change.

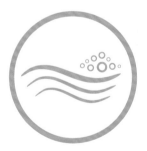

Water
Kapha energy regulates water-based functions of the body, such as urination.

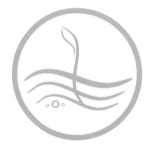

Earth
The earth element is heavy and firm, and kapha types tend to be heavily built.

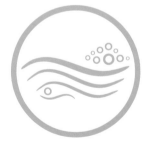

Water/earth
Kapha is made up of water and earth, and is the most reliable of the three doshas.

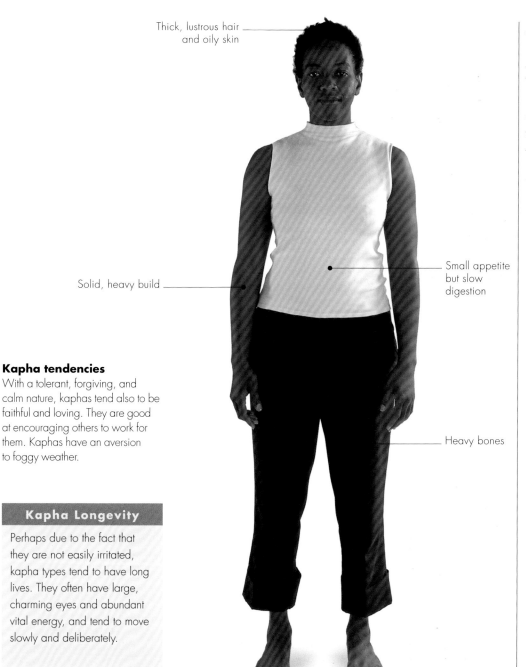

Thick, lustrous hair and oily skin

Small appetite but slow digestion

Solid, heavy build

Heavy bones

Kapha tendencies

With a tolerant, forgiving, and calm nature, kaphas tend also to be faithful and loving. They are good at encouraging others to work for them. Kaphas have an aversion to foggy weather.

Kapha Imbalances

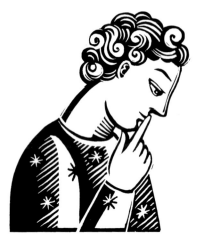

Sturdy & reliable
Kapha types are loving and secure, and they act slowly, rationally, and calmly.

Calm and serene, the kapha type has a sensitive, intuitive nature and good overall health. Heavy boned, this type has a tendency to put on weight, particularly since they have a love of good food. Kaphas rarely have trouble sleeping; in fact kaphas are prone to oversleeping. Their faithful, loving nature is sometimes due to inertia and laziness, but their love of peace, quiet, and stability in their life and surroundings is genuine.

What causes imbalance?

The main cause of imbalance in kapha types is a lack of stimulation, which can lead to inertia. Other causes of kapha imbalance include cold, damp weather, overeating, a diet that is too high in sugar, fat, or salt (sweet, sour, and salty foods aggravate kapha), insufficient exercise, and excess sleep—especially naps taken during the daytime.

Signs of balanced kapha

When balanced, this type can be delightful—a good friend, patient, compassionate, courageous, and emotionally stable. Physically, kaphas are sturdy and strong, with good joints, a solid physique, good nutritional status, high sexual potency, and good digestion. Although kaphas would prefer to avoid exercise if possible, they show greater stamina than the other doshas once they are encouraged into a routine. Kapha provides the body with its resistance to disease and also gives great support to the healing process. It is the anabolic force in the body, which means that it governs the formation of even the smallest cells. It is supportive of the mental processes that are stabilizing and strengthening, such as loyalty, forgiveness, and love.

Signs of Imbalance

All of the following symptoms, or combinations of symptoms, can be telltale signs that kapha is in a state of imbalance.

- Pale skin
- Sensitivity to cold
- Poor digestion and excess weight
- Oversleeping
- Poor metabolism
- Respiratory problems
- Edema
- Allergies
- Depression
- Jealousy
- Apathy or inertia
- Impotence

Types of Kapha

There are five types of kapha in the body. *Kledaka* is found in the stomach; *avalambaka* is found in the heart; *bodhaka* is found in the tongue; *tarpaka* is found in the head, and *sleshaka* is found in the joints. Therefore, when there is a kapha imbalance you can expect deficiencies and problems in these areas.

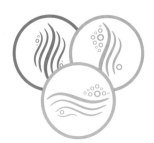

What combination?

It is very common to be more than one dosha type, although one often predominates.

WHAT'S YOUR DOSHA?
Many readers will recognize themselves in the portraits on pages 34 to 45. Your constitutional type will, however, be unique to you. There are seven main constitutional types: three in which one dosha predominates (kapha, pitta, and vata), three which reflect a strong blend of two doshas (vata/pitta, pitta/kapha, or vata/kapha), and one in which all three doshas seem to have an equal influence.

Making an assessment

The questions on the following pages are designed to help you to pinpoint your dosha. It is best to answer these questions twice—once on your own and once with a friend, who can offer their opinion, since it can be difficult to be objective about yourself. If you come up with two different answers, do the quiz again with another friend or family member.

Diagnosing the patient

A practitioner will be able to make a precise diagnosis of your type and any imbalance through checking various signs.

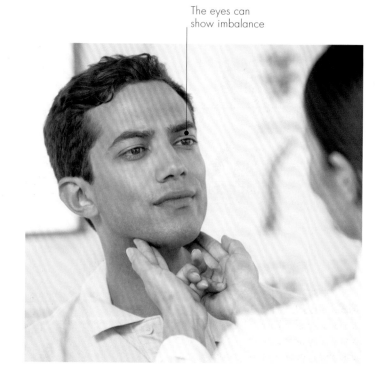

The eyes can show imbalance

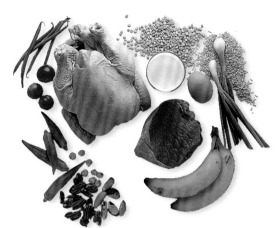

Vata foods

If you know your dosha, you can use diet to help balance it—meat is often vital in the vata diet.

Pitta foods

Pitta types should eat raw foods wherever possible, focusing on cool, refreshing foods, particularly in summer.

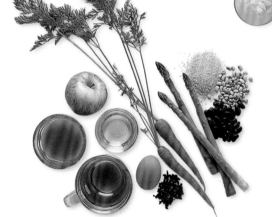

Scoring

Simply answer "yes" or "no" to the questions asked for each character type. Add up the yes answers for each type. If one type has many, many more "yes" answers than the others, you can be fairly certain that this is your dosha type. If two types seem fairly equally balanced, with a third trailing behind, your type is likely to be a combination of the first two doshas. Only rarely do people have a roughly equal balance between the three.

Kapha foods

Kapha types should eat plenty of vegetables and avoid wheat and meat. They benefit from eating mostly cooked foods.

What Type Are You?

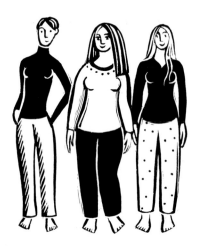

What shape are you?

Your physical appearance is one of the factors that help to define your constitutional type.

First of all, think about your physical appearance and constitution. The questions on these pages cover everything from the way you look and your body's response to its surroundings to how your system copes with food and how you sound when you speak. Run through the lists and mark the relevant boxes. It is useful to do this with a friend to reach an objective assessment. If you are not sure about an answer, continue through the list and go back to the question later on. (For Scoring, see page 47.)

Vata

- Are you very tall, or short and thin? ☐
- Is your frame light and narrow? ☐
- Are you slim, and do you find it difficult to gain weight? ☐
- Is your complexion dark? ☐
- Do you have an average amount of hair? ☐
- Are your eyes small, narrow, or sunken? ☐
- Are your eyes dark or gray? ☐
- Do your teeth protrude? ☐
- Are your teeth very small or very large? ☐
- Do you have low stamina? ☐
- Do you prefer warmth to cold? ☐
- Do you often have constipation? ☐
- Is your voice weak, low, hoarse, or quavering? ☐
- Do you speak quickly? ☐
- Do you prefer sweet, salty, heavy, or oily foods? ☐
- Is your pulse rate above 70 if you are male, and above 80 if you are female? ☐

TOTAL

Pitta

- Are you of medium height and medium musculature? ☐
- Are you of medium weight? ☐
- Do you sweat a lot when it's hot? ☐
- Is your skin soft and quite warm? ☐
- Is your complexion fair or pink? ☐
- Is your hair fine, soft, red, or fair? ☐
- Are your eyes of average size? ☐
- Are your eyes blue, gray, or hazel? ☐
- Are your teeth average in size and yellowish in color? ☐
- Do you have stamina and strength? ☐
- Do you prefer coolness to warmth? ☐
- Do your bowel movements tend to produce loose stools? ☐
- Do you talk convincingly and have precise speech? ☐
- Do you prefer sweet, light, warm, and bitter foods? ☐
- Are you usually hungry, and do you feel uncomfortable when you miss a meal? ☐
- Is your pulse 60–70 if you are male, and 70–80 if you are female? ☐

TOTAL

Kapha

- Are you solid and fairly big? ☐
- Is your frame large and broad? ☐
- Do you gain weight easily? ☐
- Do you sweat minimally? ☐
- Is your skin moist and cool? ☐
- Is your complexion pale? ☐
- Is your hair thick, lustrous, and brown? ☐
- Are your eyes large and prominent? ☐
- Are your eyes blue or brown? ☐
- Do you have white teeth and strong gums? ☐
- Do you have large teeth? ☐
- Do you move steadily but slowly? ☐
- Do you have good endurance? ☐
- Do you have normal bowel movements? ☐
- Do you have a fairly steady appetite, and an ability to skip meals easily? ☐
- Do you speak slowly? ☐
- Do you prefer dry, low-fat, sweet, and spicy foods? ☐
- Is your pulse below 60 if you are male, and below 70 if you are female? ☐

TOTAL

YOUR MIND

The next set of questions concentrates on your state of mind. Think about the way that you approach life, and consider your mental and emotional response to your surroundings. What sorts of moods do you experience? How do you approach day-to-day tasks and challenges? Once again, you should compare your own "yes" or "no" responses with the objective viewpoint of a friend. Again, if you are unsure of an answer, leave the question and go back to it later on.

Vata		Pitta		Kapha	
• Are you active?	☐	• Can you be argumentative?	☐	• Is your memory good?	☐
• Do you eat at odd times?	☐	• Do you sleep soundly, for 6–8 hours on average?	☐	• Are you complacent?	☐
• Do you become anxious?	☐			• Are you usually calm?	☐
• Is your lifestyle erratic?	☐	• Is your memory sharp?	☐	• Are you logical and stable?	☐
• Is your sleep interrupted?	☐	• Are you busy, but manage to achieve a lot in a day?	☐	• Do you sleep deeply, and need a lot of sleep?	☐
• Are you fairly fearful?	☐				
• Are you insecure?	☐	• Are you fiery and angry, and tend to be judgmental?	☐	• Do you tend toward being greedy or possessive?	☐
• Are you restless with plenty of new ideas?	☐				
• Do you have a good short-term memory?	☐	• Are you precise and logical?	☐	• Is it difficult to irritate you?	☐
• Do you react badly to stress?	☐	• Do you have a quick temper?	☐	• Is your mood fairly steady?	☐
• Are you creative?	☐	• Are you intellectual?	☐		
• Are you moody?	☐	• Do your moods tend to change slowly?	☐		
TOTAL		TOTAL		TOTAL	

Mental energy

Your constitutional type will affect the state of your memory, emotions, temperament, and even your creativity.

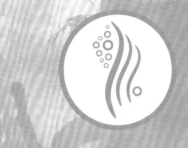

Working Out the Results

The dosha type with the greatest number of "yes" answers is your predominant constitutional type. If two types have a similar number of "yes" answers, you are probably one of the four secondary constitutional types (see page 46). For example, if you had 30 vata answers, 10 pitta answers, and 2 kapha answers, your constitutional type would be vata; if you had 20 vata answers, 20 pitta answers, and 4 kapha answers, your type would be vata/pitta.

The Mind's Constitution

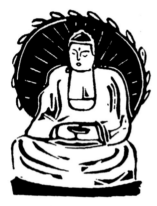

Enlightenment
*Sattvic is the purest state
of mind; good living is required
to reach this enlightenment.*

Not only are there three main
constitutional types of the body,
the three doshas, but the mind
also has its own constitution. The mind
can be either *sattvic, rajasic,* or *tamasic,*
or a combination of the three. Sattvic is the
highest and purest state of mind, when
the mind rests in equilibrium. Being fully
sattvic is very rare, but Ayurveda aims to
take everyone closer to this state of being.
Practicing meditation and living in a wise
and ethical way can help us to move
further toward it.

The three states of mind

Eating well, sleeping well, being positive,
confident, and respectful, and being a
good, kind person with an acute sense
of well-being marks out the person with
a sattvic mind.

At the other end of the scale is the
tamasic mind, which is considered to be
low and ignorant. Tamasic people can
be negative, demanding, egotistical, and
selfish, and they lack energy. They have a
poor diet and little sense of well-being.

The rajasic mind is passionate and often
angry, and rajasic people can be subject
to mood swings. They may overindulge in
everything, including sex, food, exercise,
alcohol, work, and leisure pursuits.

Reaching the sattvic state

When there is too much rajasic or tamasic
in the mind, disturbance results and the
sattvic state becomes impossible to attain.
The system of ayurveda aims to purify the
mind, body, and spirit on every level to
reach toward the sattvic state. It does this
through its detoxification therapies and
regulation of diet and lifestyle, and through

yoga, meditation, and other practices. Following the Ayurvedic principles can help to lead one further toward an enlightened state of mind.

Your Mental Constitution

Every person is endowed with all the three properties of mind—sattvic, rajasic, and tamasic—but they vary in different people, determining what's known as the *manasa prakrithi* (state of mind) of an individual. Which are you? You will need someone else to look at this with you. It can be difficult to be completely honest about ourselves.

• In general, a sattvic person is kind, benevolent, intelligent, generous, scholarlike, courageous, bold, and truthful.

• The rajasic person is generally impatient, egoistic, fidgety, fickle-minded, anxious for self-respect, ruthless, full of anger, excessively happy, indulges in an excessive sex life, and travels without any purpose.

• Similarly a tamasic individual is often full of anxiety and worry, lacking in intelligence, ignorant, easily deluded, apathetic, resistant to change, ill-tempered, and lethargic. The tamasic person is also likely to indulge in excessive sleep and in sedentary habits.

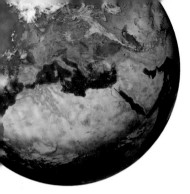

Forming the universe
The Earth, its inhabitants, and everything in the universe are formed by the five elements.

THE FIVE ELEMENTS
Ether (space), air, fire, water, and earth are also known as *panchamahabhutas*. They are present in all matter, in various proportions, and compose everything in the universe. Humans have five sense organs: ears, skin, eyes, tongue, and nose. Each is designed to perceive a form of external energy and absorb it into the body.

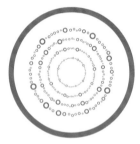

Ether/space
Vata governs ether/space.

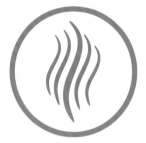

Air
Vata governs air.

Fire
Pitta governs fire.

Correspondences
The energies perceived by the five senses are the five elements. Each is created out of the others. All five exist in all things, including ourselves. In a healthy body, the five elements work in harmony, but an imbalance in any one element stimulates change in all of the others.

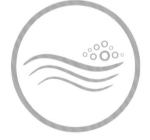

Water
Pitta and kapha govern water.

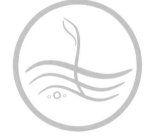

Earth
Kapha governs earth.

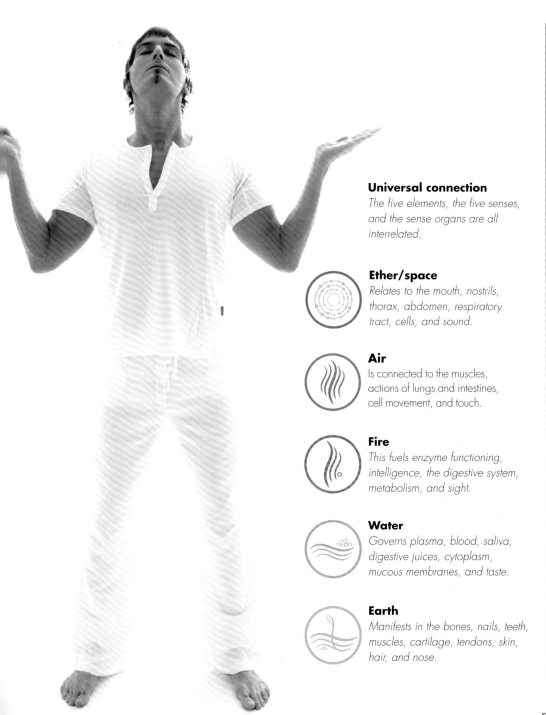

Universal connection

The five elements, the five senses, and the sense organs are all interrelated.

Ether/space

Relates to the mouth, nostrils, thorax, abdomen, respiratory tract, cells, and sound.

Air

Is connected to the muscles, actions of lungs and intestines, cell movement, and touch.

Fire

This fuels enzyme functioning, intelligence, the digestive system, metabolism, and sight.

Water

Governs plasma, blood, saliva, digestive juices, cytoplasm, mucous membranes, and taste.

Earth

Manifests in the bones, nails, teeth, muscles, cartilage, tendons, skin, hair, and nose.

The Seven Stages of Imbalance

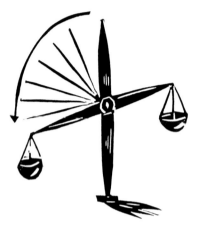

Off center

When we live stressful lives, we disrupt our innate balance, and ill health is the result.

When our energy forces become unbalanced, illness sets in. We have already discussed the various ways in which imbalance of the three doshas can occur; for example, by overworking, overtaxing our system, using our senses inappropriately, or working against our internal clocks, we can cause a condition that allows illness to develop and take hold.

Human beings are not machines. The mind, body, and spirit all need to be fed with the best possible ingredients in order to attain optimum health and well-being. When we live life on the run, burning the candle at both ends, working in a job we may not like, eating processed junk foods, smoking cigarettes, and drinking too much alcohol in order to relax, and becoming negative or stressed out, we disrupt all our body processes. This imbalance manifests itself in seven main stages:

1 Negative influences cause one or more of the doshas to build up, throwing the others out of balance;

2 As the influences continue, the doshas become more unbalanced. This second stage is called aggravation;

3 The dosha imbalance spreads from its original site, around the body. This process is called dispersion;

4 The affected dosha moves around the body and settles in inappropriate areas, causing a build-up of waste products;

5 The first mild symptoms of illness begin to appear at these sites;

6 The mild symptoms can develop into an acute illness, the type that hits you hard suddenly, but doesn't last;

7 When the causes (in other words, the outside influences) are not addressed and dealt with, the illness can become chronic (long-term).

What does Ayurveda do?

Ayurveda aims to stop the problem at or before stage four, before it becomes illness. The keyword of Ayurveda is "prevention." If outside influences are kept under control, imbalance cannot occur in the body. When treatment is successful, the life energies are restored to equilibrium and harmony and you feel vital, healthy, and full of energy.

The Aim of Ayurveda

Ayurveda, one of the oldest holistic systems of medicine in the world, aims not only to cure disease, but also to create well-being.

Governing elements
Each of the elements governs different parts and activities of the body, so any imbalance points to a particular dosha.

THE DOSHAS & THE BODY When we become ill, an Ayurvedic practitioner needs to work out which dosha (energy) has invaded the affected part of the body. Although the doshas cannot be seen, their influence can be monitored. Cells appear different according to the predominant dosha and different areas of the body are more likely to be affected by different doshas. For example, excess vata may often manifest in the skin, nervous system, colon, and large and small intestines because these areas are associated with vata energy.

Excess vata
The area of the body most affected by excess vata is the colon. Excess vata symptoms can include flatulence, constipation, indigestion, back pain, dry skin, emotional disorders, arthritis, and also circulation problems.

Excess pitta
Areas affected by excess pitta include the skin, metabolism, small intestine, eyes, liver, and the hair on the head, so the symptoms include skin disorders, premature hair loss, diarrhea, and poor elimination processes.

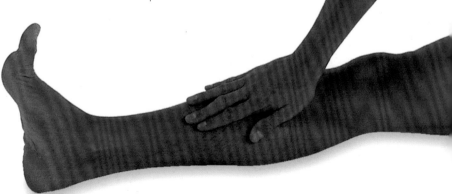

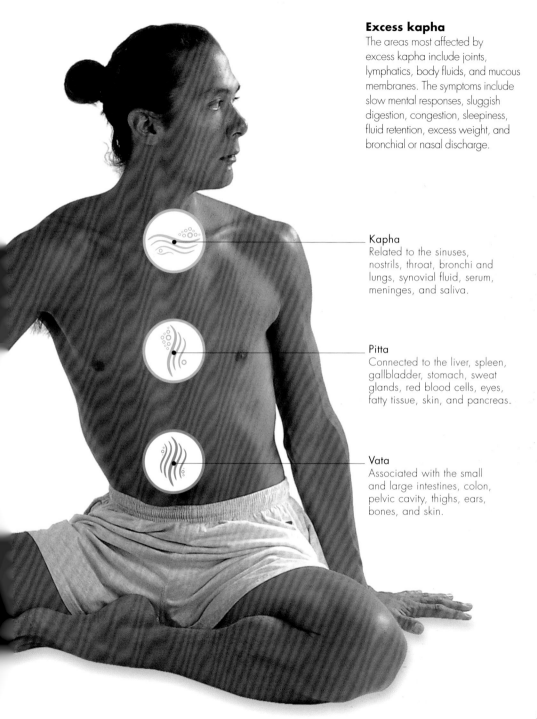

Excess kapha

The areas most affected by excess kapha include joints, lymphatics, body fluids, and mucous membranes. The symptoms include slow mental responses, sluggish digestion, congestion, sleepiness, fluid retention, excess weight, and bronchial or nasal discharge.

Kapha
Related to the sinuses, nostrils, throat, bronchi and lungs, synovial fluid, serum, meninges, and saliva.

Pitta
Connected to the liver, spleen, gallbladder, stomach, sweat glands, red blood cells, eyes, fatty tissue, skin, and pancreas.

Vata
Associated with the small and large intestines, colon, pelvic cavity, thighs, ears, bones, and skin.

The Dhaatus

Imbalance in the doshas also causes imbalance in the seven body tissues, which are known as the *dhaatus*. These are: plasma (*rasa*), blood (*raktha*), muscle (*mamsa*), fat (*madas*), bone (*asthi*), marrow and nerves (*majja*), and reproductive tissues (*shukra*). They derive energy from each other, so when one is affected, the others suffer too. Interference in the manufacture of plasma affects the quality of the blood, which affects the muscles, for example.

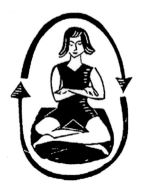

The circle of health
All of the dhaatus support and feed one another in continuous movement.

Dhaatu	Healthy	Unhealthy
RASA	Lustrous skin, vitality, joy, and a focused mind	Nausea, weakness, depression, and feelings of heaviness
RAKTHA	Sensitivity and healthy lips, feet, and nails	Inflamed vessels, abscesses, bleeding disorders, jaundice, and rashes
MAMSA	Strength and stability	Lethargy and fear
MADAS	Flexibility, honesty, and lubrication	Low vitality, numbness, and excess weight
ASTHI	Strong bones, teeth, nails, and joints, and an optimistic nature	Still joints, hair loss, and tooth decay
MAJJA	Strong immunity and joy	Bone and joint pain, fatigue, and giddiness
SHUKRA	Sexual desire, fertility, and charisma	Obsessive need for sex, period problems, and low vitality

How the dhaatus work

Each tissue type has its own process of metabolism (*agni*), which determines the metabolic changes in the tissues. Each tissue also produces by-products, which are either used in the body or excreted. Menstruation, for example, is a by-product of rasa. The tissues are also governed by the three doshas, so heavy periods can be caused by the effects of excess kapha on plasma.

The dhaatus are formed from what we eat, and by the process of agni. According to Ayurvedic wisdom, if any of these seven essential tissues becomes unbalanced, illness will result.

When the doshas are working in balance and harmony, the processes of digestion and metabolism will be efficient. If any one of the doshas is out of balance, the process will not work properly and illness will manifest itself in one of the tissues.

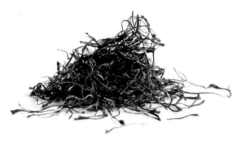

Saffron
This delicate spice is known to replenish life energy, and is used in Ayurvedic medicine.

OJAS—LIFE ENERGY
The seven dhaatus together form an energy within the body known as *ojas*. Ojas is the ultimate vital energy distilled from the dhaatus. It is located in the heart chakra (see page 91)—according to ancient Ayurvedic wisdom, eight drops of ojas are located at the heart, although strictly speaking it has no form and pervades and animates the entire body and mind. When it is nourished, there is life; when it is destroyed, we die. Where it is weakened in a specific part of the body, illness sets in; when it is built up again, healing takes place. Some practitioners consider ojas to be the fundamental energy of the immune system.

The cause of illness
There are many conditions for which Western medical practitioners can find no cause and cannot, therefore, treat. Ayurvedic practitioners believe that these conditions are the result of reduced levels of ojas. Some of these conditions include Crohn's disease, cancer, and AIDS.

Ojas & theja
Ojas, the ultimate energy, is transformed into *theja*, which refers to personal levels of energy. If there is strong theja, you will have a strong life force and high stamina. Lower levels of theja present themselves as overall weakness and a predisposition to illness.

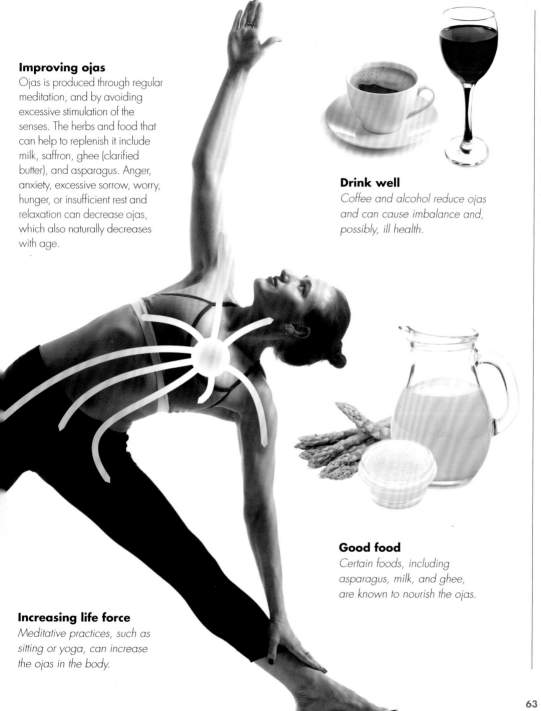

Improving ojas

Ojas is produced through regular meditation, and by avoiding excessive stimulation of the senses. The herbs and food that can help to replenish it include milk, saffron, ghee (clarified butter), and asparagus. Anger, anxiety, excessive sorrow, worry, hunger, or insufficient rest and relaxation can decrease ojas, which also naturally decreases with age.

Drink well

Coffee and alcohol reduce ojas and can cause imbalance and, possibly, ill health.

Good food

Certain foods, including asparagus, milk, and ghee, are known to nourish the ojas.

Increasing life force

Meditative practices, such as sitting or yoga, can increase the ojas in the body.

The Malas

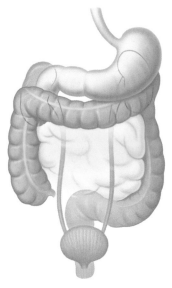

Good elimination
The efficient production and excretion of the malas is crucial for good health.

The malas are the products of the body's elimination system: sweat, urine, and feces. Body waste serves many purposes vital to healthy functioning. For example, sweating is cleansing, and helps to normalize body temperature, the urinary system removes toxins (the analysis of urine helps with diagnosis), and the steady passage of feces is essential to maintain muscle tone in the intestines.

Maintaining health

Ayurveda considers the elimination of waste products to be a crucially important part of good health. The malas flow from three main channels in the body and each has a key role:

The urinary system (which eliminates urine, or *mootra*) excretes waste through the kidneys and bladder. It also helps to maintain a healthy electrolyte balance (referring to the level of electrically charged particles in the blood) and to regulate blood pressure. Inefficient elimination of urine can cause abdominal edema (swelling), a burning sensation during urination, inflammation, and infections of the bladder and kidneys.

The fecal elimination system (which eliminates feces, or *shakrit* or *pureesha*) begins at the top of the large intestine and ends at the anus. It is also responsible for the absorption of minerals from the colon. The earth element converts food residue into a form that can be eliminated by the colon, and this process is controlled by vata energy. If waste matter is not eliminated, it will be absorbed back into the system, causing a variety of complaints, including osteoarthritis, bronchitis, asthma, lower back pain, headaches, bad breath, acne, and other "toxic" conditions.

The sweat system (which eliminates sweat, or *sweda*) deals with the production and excretion of sweat through the sweat glands. It also deals with water balance, liquid waste removal, body temperature, and skin lubrication. An inability to sweat causes dry skin and burning sensations, and essential detoxification may not take place. Ayurvedic therapy involves "sweat therapy" in order to detoxify and relieve many health conditions.

Ama

Another type of digestive waste, an accumulation of toxic chemicals, is known as *ama*. It results from an unhealthy diet and lifestyle, poor detoxification and elimination, and a high intake of toxins. The body cannot eliminate ama, and when it accumulates, it always creates disease.

THE AYURVEDIC APPROACH

The health of your body involves finding the natural, harmonious balance between the three doshas that make up your physical *prakruthi* (balanced state). A healthy mind will maintain your individual dosha balance, and good spiritual health will keep the balance between *sattva*, *rajas*, and *tamasin*. The Ayurvedic paradigm shows us how the interactions between body, mind, and spirit can be predicted, balanced, and improved, to enable us to live gracefully, harmoniously, and vigorously.

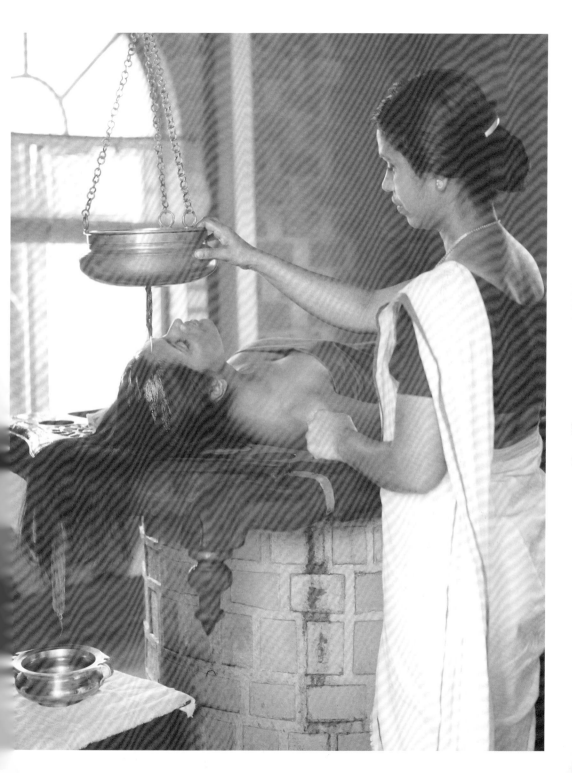

Ayurvedic Treatments

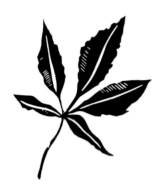

Natural therapy
Ayurvedic medicines and therapies are based on fresh, natural ingredients.

In Ayurveda, a practitioner will offer four main forms of treatment: panchakarma, medicines, dietary regimes, and regulation of lifestyle. You may also be offered or taught one or more of a wide range of therapies under the Ayurvedic umbrella.

Panchakarma

The internal detoxification program of panchakarma (see pages 72–75) aims to purify body and mind. It is usually preceded by *purvakarma*, a cleansing program involving sweat therapy and massage (see pages 70–71). These therapies are widely used in Ayurveda.

Massage & oils

Ayurvedic practitioners are trained in various forms of massage, and it is also important to include self-massage (see pages 82–85) in your day. Both dry and oil massages are used, depending on your symptoms. Plant oils are used to affect physical, mental, and emotional processes and are administered in various ways, from massage to enemas.

Marma therapy

All over the body are points through which *prana* (vital energy—see page 81) flows, maintaining well-being. Marma therapy works on these points, but should be only be offered by trained practitioners.

Herbalism

Herbal therapy, or *samana*, involves using the medicinal and energetic properties of plants to treat illness and balance the doshas. Treatments are available in various forms (see pages 94–101).

Diet

Digestion and diet are crucial to well-being in Ayurveda, and different doshas follow different diets (see pages 150–89).

Rejuvenation therapy

This type of therapy, *rasayana*, improves memory and helps to boost the body's immune system. It is also an effective way to boost your general vitality (see pages 102–5).

Routines

Seasonal routines, *ritucharya*, and daily routines, *dinacharya*, are important in Ayurveda, and you will be encouraged follow them (see pages 132–41).

Spiritual Healing

Ayurveda is aimed at the spirit as well as the body and mind, and encompasses practices such as yoga, meditation, and mantras.

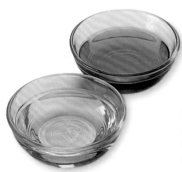

Massage
Ayurvedic massage using therapeutic oils is part of the purvakarma treatment.

PURVAKARMA
Panchakarma, a multiple-stage purification program, is the main detoxification therapy (see pages 72–75). However, purvakarma prepares the body for panchakarma therapies and is the first cleansing treatment offered to almost all patients. There are two aspects to purvakarma: massage with oils (*snehana karma*) and sweat therapy (*swedana karma*). Because massage aids the detoxification process, it forms a major part of Ayurvedic treatment.

Snehana
In this technique, herbal oils are massaged into the skin to encourage the elimination of toxins. Blended oils are used to treat specific disorders such as stress, anxiety, insomnia, arthritis, or circulation problems. Oils can also be massaged into the scalp for depression, insomnia, and memory problems. Snehana can sometimes involve lying in an oil bath, thought to be even more effective because it allows you to absorb the properties of the oils.

Swedana
Sweat therapy is sometimes used in conjunction with the oil treatment, but on a separate day. Steam baths are used to encourage the elimination of toxins through the pores. Together with the oil treatments, they make the detoxification process more effective. You may need a series of steam baths in order to remove all the toxins through the sweat.

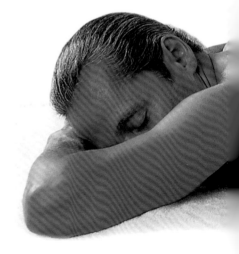

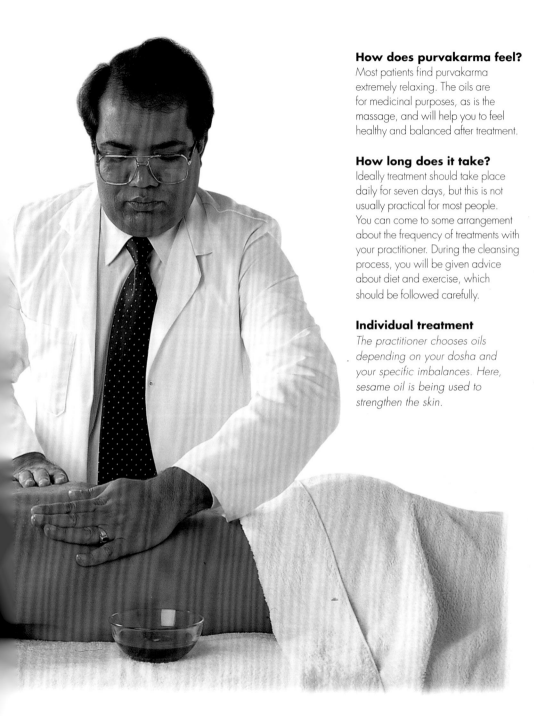

How does purvakarma feel?

Most patients find purvakarma extremely relaxing. The oils are for medicinal purposes, as is the massage, and will help you to feel healthy and balanced after treatment.

How long does it take?

Ideally treatment should take place daily for seven days, but this is not usually practical for most people. You can come to some arrangement about the frequency of treatments with your practitioner. During the cleansing process, you will be given advice about diet and exercise, which should be followed carefully.

Individual treatment

The practitioner chooses oils depending on your dosha and your specific imbalances. Here, sesame oil is being used to strengthen the skin.

The Five Therapies of Panchakarma

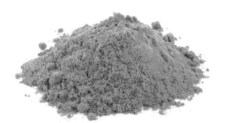

Curing with spices
Many spices, including ginger and turmeric, are used in purification processes.

Purvakarma prepares the body for the full detoxification process—panchakarma. This is a five-fold therapy, but only rarely are all five aspects used in treatment. Usually just one or two are chosen.

Virechana

This purgation therapy is used to eliminate excess pitta dosha from the small intestine. It involves taking a purgative substance and/or gentle laxative to eliminate the pitta and cleanse the blood, liver, spleen, small intestine, and sweat glands. Herbs used for virechana include senna leaf, aloe vera, dandelion, and psyllium seed.

Basti

Medicated-oil and herbal enemas, douches, and eyewashes are used in basti therapy mostly to reduce excess vata, although they can also help with pitta and kapha disorders. Vata is located in the colon, rectum, and bones, and regulates the elimination of waste products. Basti can treat constipation, lower back pain, arthritis, anxiety, headaches, viruses, and more.

Raktamokshana

This involves removing a little blood to eliminate toxins and excess pitta from the blood, lymph, and tissues. This therapy is used less often than it used to be, and herbal blood purifiers, such as yellow dock, cleavers, and turmeric, can be used instead. Conditions that respond include eczema, acne, fevers, urticaria, gout, jaundice, hemorrhoids, and genital herpes.

Vamana

Therapeutic vomiting, involving the ingesting of herbal or salty liquids, is a treatment for respiratory and congestive problems, but it is rarely used today.

Nasya

Medicines are applied through the nostrils to treat many problems, including kapha conditions of the ear, eyes, nose, and throat, and of migraine and neuralgia. Substances used include gotu kola and ginger powders, sesame oil, milk, and ghee. It is not advised for use during pregnancy and menstruation.

Nasya

When nasya is applied properly, it has a stimulating effect on the lining of the nose, causing the patient to feel light-headed.

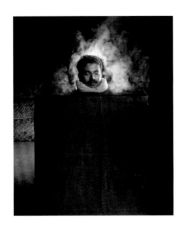

Opening the pores
Patients may sit in a closed-in steam bath as a preparation for panchakarma treatments.

BODY CLEANSING
The word *panchakarma* means "the five actions" and refers to the Ayurvedic cleansing therapies that enliven the body's own natural mechanisms for eliminating toxins from the body. They are also given to remove excess dosha energies, and to keep the doshas in check to prevent problems. Ayurveda suggests that everyone undergo a cleansing therapy at the turn of each season to eliminate excess energies accumulated during the previous season.

Shodana
Together panchakarma and purvakarma constitute *shodana*, or the "cleansing" therapies. They are seen as primary pillars of Ayurvedic treatment. Purvakarma involves oiling and sweating, to encourage the "wandering" doshas to move out of the tissues in which they have established themselves and return to their main site. From there they can be removed using panchakarma.

Internal oiling
Ayurveda suggests drinking plenty of ghee and other liquids before panchakarma.

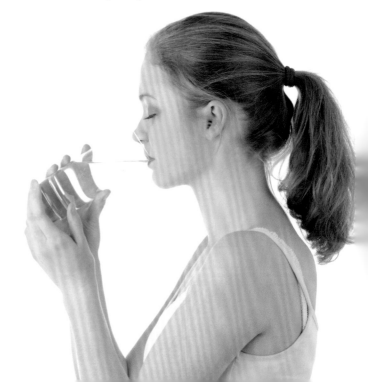

Detoxification
*Certain foods are known
to encourage the process of
detoxification, which keeps
the doshas balanced.*

Preparation
Purvakarma involves internal and
external oiling. Internal oiling is
undertaken by adding an increasing
amount of ghee to the diet over a
couple of days. The external oiling
is normally in the form of a massage,
using the appropriate oils (see
pages 80–81). The "lubrication"
encourages the dosha energies
into the circulation.

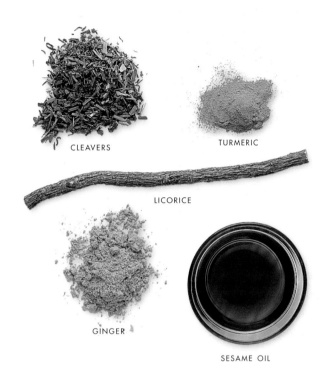

CLEAVERS

TURMERIC

LICORICE

GINGER

SESAME OIL

GHEE

SENNA
LEAVES

RHUBARB

Herbal steam bath
A steam bath with herbs also helps
to perform this task by opening the
pores, heating and liquefying the
ama (toxins), and moving it from the
tissues into the circulatory system.
When this is done, the body is
ready for panchakarma treatment,
which is the proper and effective
detoxification.

Five steps
*Rhubarb, senna leaves, and ghee
are among the natural substances
that can be used to eliminate toxins
from the body and remove excess
dosha energy.*

Ayurvedic Oil Massage

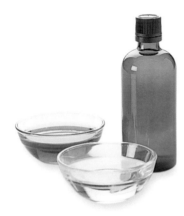

Oils for all
*Massage with oil is a key part
of Ayurvedic treatment and can
also be done at home.*

Ayurvedic oil massage has now become fashionable in the West. Various oils processed with herbs are used in Ayurveda for curing ailments ranging from insomnia to paralysis. Ayurvedic massage is also said to minimize the effects of old age. There are four types of Ayurvedic massage: *abhyanga*, *pizzichil*, *chavutti thirumal*, and *dhara*.

Abhyanga
This whole-body massage is given with different types of oils, depending on the constitution of the body and mind. The massage is performed with a combination of strokes including kneading, tapping, rubbing, touching, shaking, moving, and squeezing. Abhyanga massage is given prior to a herbal steam bath. It is useful for general rejuvenation, fatigue, body aches and musculoskeletal problems, as well as mental stress.

Pizzichil
Oil is continuously dripped onto the body from pieces of cloth dipped in oil. Normally four masseurs are required to give this massage, two to squeeze the oil from the cloths onto the patient and two to do the massaging. Pizzichil is prescribed for paralysis, motor neurone disease, multiple sclerosis, myopathy, and rheumatism.

Chavutti thirumal
In this specialized massage, one masseur hangs from the ceiling by hooks and carries out massage with the soles of the feet while others pour oil over the patient. This massage is prescribed for musculoskeletal pains, chronic fatigue syndrome, and other nervous disorders.

Dhara

This treatment involves the flow of liquids, including oils, buttermilk, coconut water, cow's milk, or decoctions of herbs and medicated oils, onto the body. It is recommended for psychosomatic disorders.

Benefits of Massage

Among its many benefits, regular Ayurvedic massage is said to:

- Strengthen nerves and improve circulation

- Regulate the digestive system

- Strengthen muscles, bones, and blood vessels

- Reduce the effects of the aging process

- Eliminate fatigue

- Improve eyesight

- Induce good sleep

- Strengthen the skin

- Improve the complexion

- Increase resistance to disease and injuries

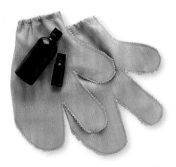

Tender touch

Using raw silk gloves to massage the body stimulates the circulation and metabolism.

MASSAGE

Massage is one of the best ways to encourage the flow of energy in the body and the release of toxins and waste, and regular treatments are encouraged in Ayurveda. Massaging the skin stimulates blood circulation and encourages the flow of lymph, speeding up the elimination of *ama*, or toxins. When vegetable oil is massaged into the skin, it offers an immediate source of nutrition for the body.

Dry massage

Dry massage is extremely stimulating, particularly for the connective tissues, circulation, and metabolism, and is especially useful in treating those who are overweight. It is also recommended when you are recovering from an illness or a course of medical treatment. Use raw silk gloves when dry massaging yourself. They can be found in pharmacies or specialist Ayurvedic suppliers. Massage for four or five minutes only—never any longer—preferably first thing in the morning. Follow treatment with a warm bath, to encourage the toxins and waste products to leave the body.

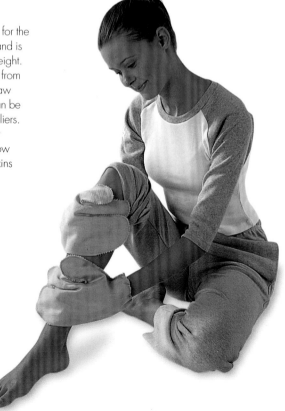

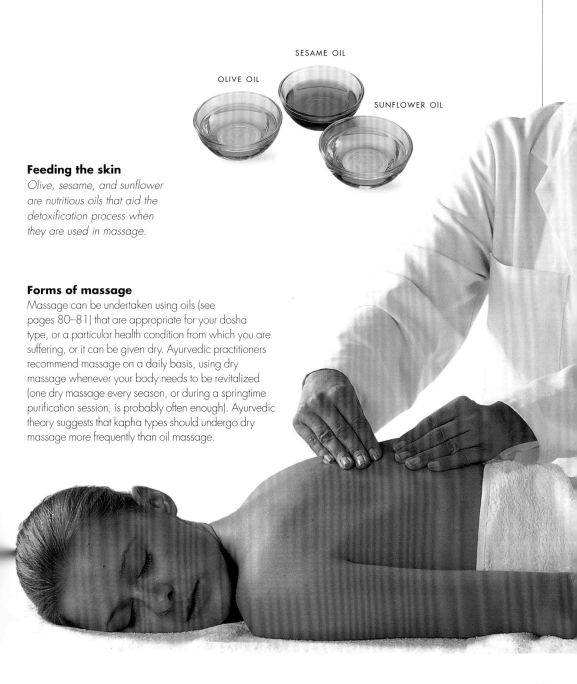

SESAME OIL

OLIVE OIL

SUNFLOWER OIL

Feeding the skin

*Olive, sesame, and sunflower
are nutritious oils that aid the
detoxification process when
they are used in massage.*

Forms of massage

Massage can be undertaken using oils (see
pages 80–81) that are appropriate for your dosha
type, or a particular health condition from which you are
suffering, or it can be given dry. Ayurvedic practitioners
recommend massage on a daily basis, using dry
massage whenever your body needs to be revitalized
(one dry massage every season, or during a springtime
purification session, is probably often enough). Ayurvedic
theory suggests that kapha types should undergo dry
massage more frequently than oil massage.

Using Massage

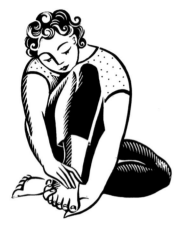

Self-massage
*Depending on your dosha type,
you will need to self-massage
more or less frequently.*

Oil massage is recommended for most dosha types on a regular basis. Vata types should self-massage once a day, as part of their morning routine, while kapha and pitta types should massage only two or three times a week. Following the massage, the oils should be left on the body for between 15 and 35 minutes, and then a warm, herbal steam or hot bath is recommended for 20 to 40 minutes more. The purpose of the bath is not just to remove the oils—sweat therapy is an essential part of the detoxification process. A great deal of waste can be eliminated through the skin, and sweating keeps the pores open and the skin soft.

Which oil?

Different oils are recommended for the different dosha types. For example, the best oil to use for vata types is good-quality, cold-pressed sesame oil, which strengthens the skin and protects it from fungal infections and the harmful effects of the sun. If you find that this irritates your skin, use olive oil or sweet almond oil instead. Clarified butter (ghee) can also be used. Always heat the oil to body temperature before using it. Many more oils can be used, but the recommendations below are a good selection for your daily massage.

Vata types Choose calming oils, including sesame, olive, almond, wheat germ, and castor oil.

Pitta types Choose cooling oils, such as coconut, sandalwood, pumpkin seed, almond, and sunflower oil.

Kapha types Choose burning oils. These include mustard, corn, and safflower oils.

Encouraging energy

According to Ayurveda, many of us hold our bodies in unnatural postures which limit the free flow of prana (vital energy). A whole-body massage helps to ensure that the marma points, through which prana flows, are addressed (see pages 86–89). Before massage, lie quietly for a few moments and breathe deeply, in order to unwind and relax.

After your bath, try to lie down for a little while. Avoid stimulants, such as caffeine, for the first few hours, and try to keep calm. Don't take physical exercise or expose yourself to extreme cold. The massage will leave you in a fragile, peaceful frame of mind, and you do not want to destroy that serenity.

After Massage

Don't forget that oil is very slippery, so enter and leave the bath carefully. Wear cotton socks to avoid marking carpets and bedding.

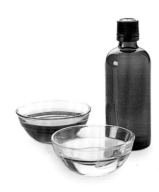

Natural oils
Choose natural oils for massaging to encourage the good health of your skin.

TEN-MINUTE SELF-MASSAGE
Ayurvedic full-body massage is called *abhyanga*, and apart from its various therapeutic benefits, listed on page 77, it provides the body with nourishment and vitality. It is quite easy to give yourself a therapeutic massage, and 10 to15 minutes is sufficient for a quick treatment. By moving the energies throughout the body, a daily massage will leave you feeling invigorated and balanced, keeping toxins at a low level and encouraging overall good health.

Preparation
Sit on a low stool or on the floor, on a warm towel. Ensure that your bathroom or whichever room you choose is warm and free from drafts. Apply the warm oil all over your body and wait a few minutes for it to become absorbed before you begin the self-massage.

Massage sequence
1 *Use gentle, circular movements, complemented by upward and downward strokes with the heel of your hand. Repeat each movement three times as the oil is smoothed into your skin.*

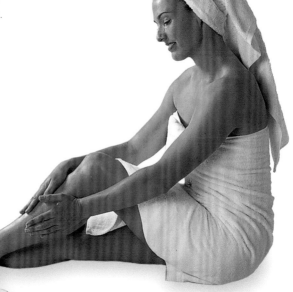

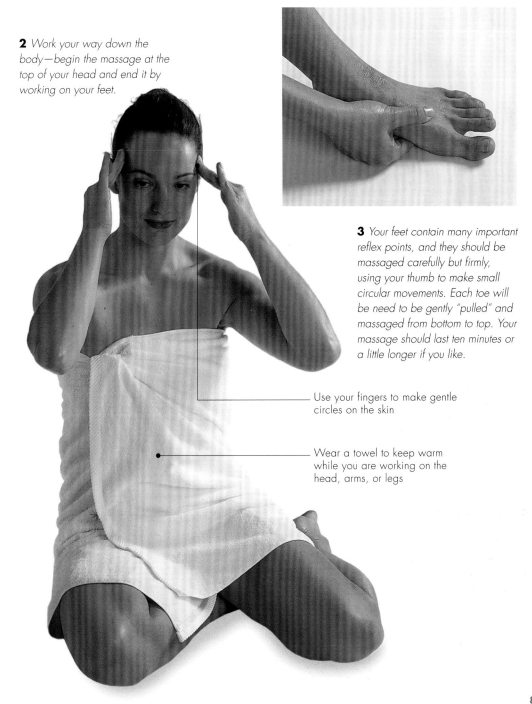

2 *Work your way down the body—begin the massage at the top of your head and end it by working on your feet.*

3 *Your feet contain many important reflex points, and they should be massaged carefully but firmly, using your thumb to make small circular movements. Each toe will be need to be gently "pulled" and massaged from bottom to top. Your massage should last ten minutes or a little longer if you like.*

Use your fingers to make gentle circles on the skin

Wear a towel to keep warm while you are working on the head, arms, or legs

83

Self-massage for the Body

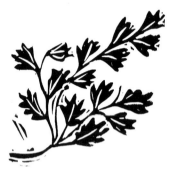

Simple healing
Gentle strokes and soothing oils offer a natural, wholesome way to improve your well-being.

The entire body benefits from Ayurvedic self-massage, and it is important to address every area with the oils and massage strokes. If you are older or suffer from circulatory disorders, speak to your doctor before massaging. Ayurveda also recommends that you avoid massage during the first three days of your period. Massage is fine if you are pregnant, but choose your oils with care—most general books on aromatherapy will tell you which oils to avoid. Warm oil is much more pleasant to use than cold oil, and it sinks gently into the skin.

Massage routine

Follow the preparation instructions on page 82. Use your fingertips to massage your scalp, as though washing your hair. Start at the hairline and work over the sides of your head to your neck. Massage the edges and lobes of your ears and move onto your forehead, moving your fingers outward toward your temples. Massage the temples with a small, circular motion.

Massage your cheeks and chin, and across your nose. Move to your neck and throat. Lay one hand on each shoulder blade, then stroke up toward the roots of your hair.

Massage your right arm first, then your left, using firm upward and downward strokes and circular strokes for the joints. Hold each finger out and stroke it toward the nail.

Massage your chest with gentle, circular movements. Women should massage around their breasts, using upward and downward strokes along the breastbone. Stroke your abdomen with circular, clockwise movements. Massage in ever-increasing circles, using only a little pressure. You will need to stand for the next part of this routine. Massage your back and buttocks with the palms of your hands in an upward and downward movement. Gently massage the genitals, paying particular attention to the area between the perineum and the anus.

Massage your legs in the same way as you massaged your arms, first the right leg and then the left. Use circular movements for knee and ankle joints.

For your feet, start at the tips of the toes and work upward toward the ankle. Then repeat the process back out to the ends of your toes. Use your thumbs to massage the soles of your feet, pressing in with small spiral movements from the heel to the toes. Squeeze each toe individually, and massage between them.

Caution

If you suffer from skin, circulation, or immune system problems, you should see your doctor before beginning a self-massage program.

MARMA POINTS

The marma points relate to different doshas and can be used to ease symptoms of ill health. Here, green denotes vata, orange is pitta, and blue is kapha.

Back Marma Points

Arms
1 Wrist injuries, inflammations, stiff finger joints
3 Wrist injuries, inflammations, stiff finger joints
5 Wrist injuries, inflammations, mental problems
7 Stiff elbow, liver, spleen, and pancreas problems
11 Pain in neck and shoulder, numbness in hands, stiff fingers

Legs
2 Pain in feet, leg injuries, dropped arches
3 Ankle injuries, swelling, arthritis
6 Muscle cramps in calf, varicose veins

Back
1 Hemorrhoids, rectal prolapse, constipation
2 Arthritis in hip, injury to hip
3 Sciatica, pain or muscle cramps in leg, arthritis in hip
4 Sacroiliac joint problems, lumbar back pain, sciatica, reproductive organs
5 Low back pain, stiff back
6 Circulation problems, shoulder and neck pain, headaches
7 Stiff neck, neck injuries, headaches
8 Shoulder pain, injury, muscle cramps in shoulder blade
9 Weakness in hands, paralysis, numbness

Head & neck
4 Stiff neck, headache, neck injury, stammering
5 Dizziness, vertigo, deafness, inflammation in ear
12 Headaches, convulsions, epilepsy, memory loss
14 Headache, migraine, memory loss, lack of energy

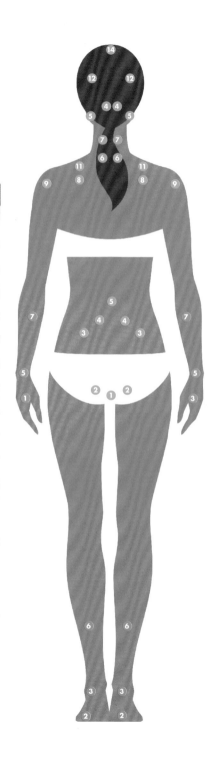

Front Marma Points

Arms

2 Wrist injuries, inflammations, stiff finger joints, heart problems
4 Wrist injuries, inflammations, stiff finger joints
6 Tennis elbow, stiff elbow
8 Cramps in upper arm
9 Poor circulation of blood to hand, muscle cramps
10 Poor circulation of blood to hand, muscle cramps

Legs

1 Poor circulation to feet and legs, numbness, foot injuries
4 Ankle and foot injuries, arthritis, edema
5 Ankle problems, arthritis, reproductive problems
7 Knee injuries, arthritis, edema
8 Cramps in calf muscles
9 Pain and cramps in thigh, poor circulation
10 Poor leg circulation, leg cramps
11 Infertility, constipation, hernia, menstrual problems

Trunk

1 Prostate problems, cystitis, reproductive problems
2 Constipation, diarrhea, colic, indigestion
3 Heart disease, blood pressure/circulation problems
4 Mastitis, tender breasts
5 Mastitis, swollen breasts
6 Shoulder cramps, injuries, breathing problems
7 Bronchitis, asthma, breathing problems, panic attacks

Head & neck

1 Headache, speech difficulty, paralysis
2 Stammering, paralysis, sore throat, thyroid problems
3 Stiff neck, speech problems, throat infections
6 Loss of sense of smell, congestion, rhinitis, nasal polyp
7 Trigeminal neuralgia, headache, facial paralysis
8 Migraine, vertigo, loss of hearing, loss of memory
9 Migraine, vertigo, loss of memory
10 Migraine, headaches, vertigo
11 Loss of smell, congestion, pituitary problems
13 Sinusitis, frontal headache
15 Anxiety and depression

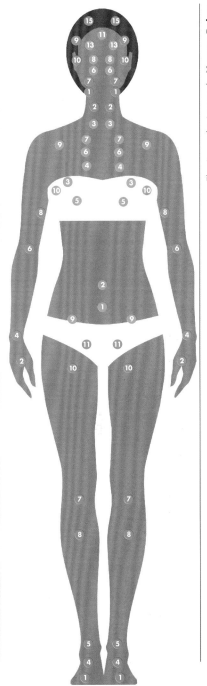

The Marmas

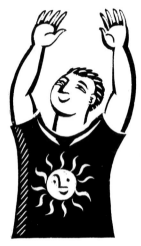

Flowing energy
*Stimulating the marma
points affects the chakras and
helps energy to flow freely
through the body.*

In order to be healthy, our natural, vital
life energy must be able to flow freely
throughout the channels of our body.
This life energy, or prana, can become
blocked or stagnant when our bodies are
injured, when we adopt chronically poor
posture, when we experience emotional
blocks or traumas, and when we suffer
illnesses or diseases that affect the flow
of prana throughout the body.

What are marma points?

Marma points are positions on the body
where flesh, veins, arteries, tendons, and
bones meet. They may be seen as the
junctions where vata, pitta, and kapha,
or sattiva, rajas, and tamas, meet, or even
where eternity and relativity meet. They
are points that have great importance
to a person's body, mind, and spirit.

Ayurveda details major and minor
marma points. Major points correspond to
the chakras (see pages 90–93) and minor
points are found around the torso, limbs,
and head area. Because marma points are
the nodal points where life force is situated,
they are very sensitive. *Mamsa marmas*
are vulnerable muscles, *sira marmas*
are vulnerable veins, *asthi marmas* are
vulnerable points on bones, and *sandhi
marmas* are vulnerable points on joints.

There are 107 nodal points, 12 of
which, including the head, heart, and
bladder, are very important. If they are
injured, serious harm to the body (and
even death) can result. Because of this,
it is important that you accept marma
therapy only from very experienced
practitioners (see box, right).

Using the marma points

Marma therapy, which involves applying
pressure to the points with or without
needles, affects the physical body, chakras,
and doshas. Its aim is to stimulate bodily
organs and systems. Marma points
are similar to those used in Chinese
acupuncture, but many are larger and
can be found more easily.

Marma is discussed in one of the four
main Vedas, and detailed in the classical
Ayurvedic text *Sushrut Samhita*. It is
possible that Chinese acupuncture was
developed after texts describing marma
therapy were taken to China.

Caution

Marma therapy should be practiced only by
qualified Ayurvedic physicians with recognized
university degrees and who have had a number
of years' experience under marma experts. While
marma therapy can cure illness effectively, incorrect
practice can be dangerous and even fatal.

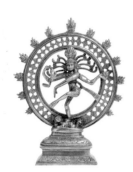

Spiritual energy
Working on the chakras is a practice that requires the guidance of a spiritual master.

THE CHAKRAS
Chakras are centers of energy that are located along the midline of the body, in line with the spinal cord. There are seven chakras, and these are related to the main marma points (see pages 86–89), which receive energy generated by the chakras. The seven chakras affect our physical existence, our physiology, our emotions, and our spiritual progression.

Imagining the chakras
Chakras are envisaged as lotus flowers, creating a channel through the body, from the base of the spine to just above the head. A type of energy called *kundalini* moves from the lowest to the highest chakra as we travel along the path to spirituality and divine knowledge.

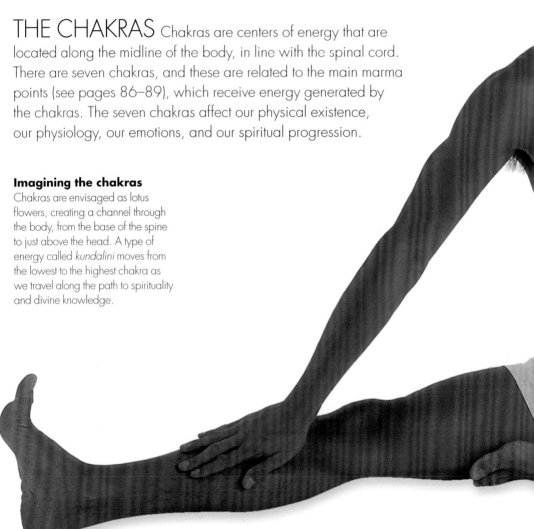

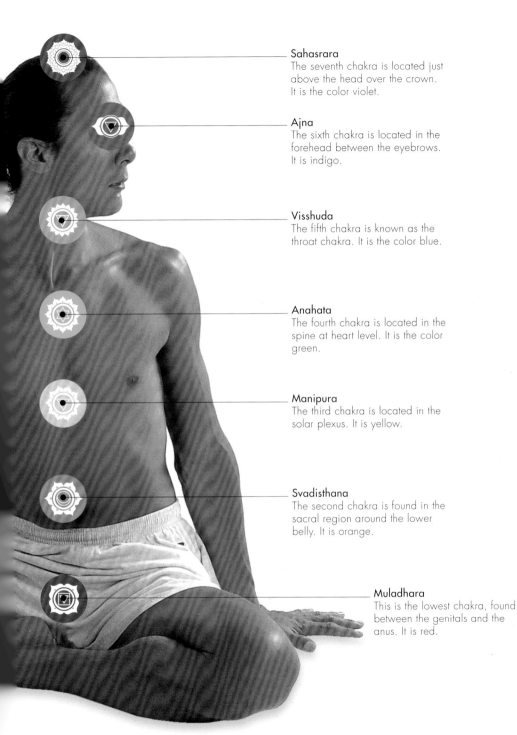

Sahasrara
The seventh chakra is located just above the head over the crown. It is the color violet.

Ajna
The sixth chakra is located in the forehead between the eyebrows. It is indigo.

Visshuda
The fifth chakra is known as the throat chakra. It is the color blue.

Anahata
The fourth chakra is located in the spine at heart level. It is the color green.

Manipura
The third chakra is located in the solar plexus. It is yellow.

Svadisthana
The second chakra is found in the sacral region around the lower belly. It is orange.

Muladhara
This is the lowest chakra, found between the genitals and the anus. It is red.

Working with the Chakras

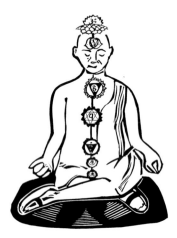

Meditation

A regular meditation practice can help energy to move up through the chakras.

Western scientists have confirmed that the chakras correspond to the pathways of the brain and the immune system, and many Westernized health gurus offer techniques for opening the chakras in an attempt to balance energy and improve well-being.

The idea is that when these powerful energy centers are clear, good health and well-being will result, and a state of bliss can be achieved.

A spiritual practice

A reputable Ayurvedic practitioner will explain that opening the chakras is a process of evolution that can take many lifetimes, and this practice should be undertaken only in the hands of a spiritually trained guide. It is important to note that opening or unblocking the chakras is a potentially dangerous concept and it can lead to serious mental problems.

However, what you can do is to work with a practitioner, using yoga and/or meditation, in order to focus on specific chakras that relate to marma points—in other words, you can use physical, mental, and spiritual techniques to move kundalini energy from points at which it has become blocked or stagnant. In this case, the aim is not to work upward through the chakras in a conscious process toward spiritual enlightenment, but to focus instead on areas of the body where energy is not moving.

Color visualization

A knowledge of the seven chakras is useful when you are trying to move blocked energy from an area of the body.

Each chakra is related to different parts of the body, and has its own color (see page 91). Visualizing and focusing on the color of the appropriate chakra while you are meditating can help to address problems relating to that area of the body. For example, working on the fourth chakra may help to ease problems of the heart on both the physiological and emotional levels.

Chakras in Ayurveda

Chakra therapy as such is not part of Ayurvedic medicine, although it can form part of a spiritual program. In addition, a knowledge of the positions of the seven chakras can help with the spiritual healing of physical and emotional ailments. However, Ayurvedic practitioners recommend that you work on the chakras only under the guidance of a spiritual teacher.

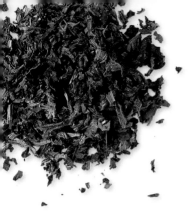

Comfrey
Comfrey is a commonly used herb, which is often prescribed to pitta types.

HERBAL REMEDIES
Ayurvedic herbalism is known as *samana*, and herbs are prescribed to correct imbalances in the doshas. These stimulate *agni* (the digestive fire, or metabolism) and restore the balance between the doshas. Herbs are not prescribed to eradicate disease because disease is just a symptom of dosha imbalance. Ayurveda has a long and honorable tradition of using herbal medicine. Under the umbrella of samana, minerals and other natural substances may be prescribed, although the use of these depends upon where Ayurveda is being practiced.

The treatment process
Treatment normally takes place across three to six months. There may be a break in herbal treatment, to give the body a rest, after which it will be resumed. *Anupana* is the Sanskrit term for "carrier substance," and this is an important part of Ayurvedic herbal treatment. When taken prior to treatment, the anupana will encourage the remedies to travel to the correct site within the body. Commonly used anupanas are honey, ghee, warm water, and milk.

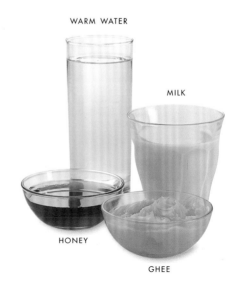

WARM WATER

MILK

HONEY

GHEE

Tailored remedies

There are many hundreds of remedies in Ayurvedic herbalism which will be selected according to your constitution and whatever condition is affecting you.

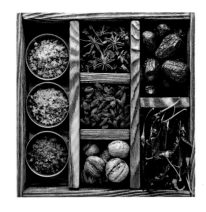

The action of herbs

Herbs can have many effects on the body, including purifying the blood, binding stools, aiding digestion, expelling worms, healing fractures, improving coagulation, increasing appetite, lowering fever, reducing toxins, balancing the tridosha or increasing or decreasing the three doshas, and strengthening the heart.

Which herb?

A full case history is normally taken before any Ayurvedic herbs are prescribed.

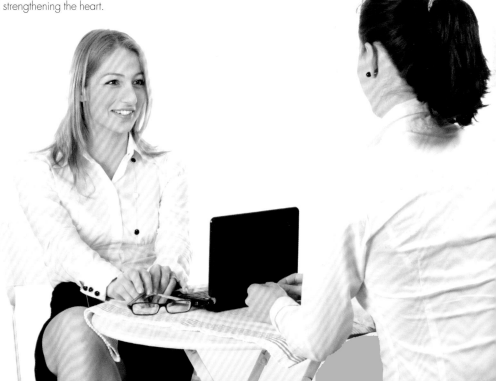

Herbalism in Practice

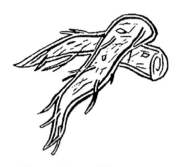

Natural nourishment
*Apart from their therapeutic
qualities, herbs are prescribed
for their nutritional benefits.*

After detoxification (see pages
70–75), your practitioner may
prescribe herbal or mineral
remedies to correct imbalances in the
doshas. Herbal remedies are usually
prescribed in liquid form or as dried
herbs, although they can also come
in powder form or tablet form.

Herbal combinations

Herbs are often taken in conjunction
with others, to work synergistically. In
combination, many herbs have an effect
greater than the sum of their separate
actions. Your constitutional type and
any dosha imbalances will be important
factors in deciding what herbs are
chosen. There are also many other factors
to consider, including the properties and
tastes of the plant (see pages 158–61),
and the time that it takes to grow. The
ingredients are pre-prepared, but different
blends are prescribed for the individual.
Each ingredient is classified by the
effect it has on lowering or increasing
levels of the dosha.

The properties of herbs

In many cases, the whole plant is used
in an Ayurvedic treatment; in others only
one part is used. All plants are described
in terms of their *rasas* (the tastes) and
gunas (the properties).

Every plant contains one or more of
the six basic tastes: sweet, acidic, salty,
pungent, bitter, and astringent (see page
160). The gunas (the properties) are
distinctive characteristics that stem from
the belief that everything in the universe
is made up of opposites. There are 20
gunas, which are hot and cold, hard and
soft, oily and dry, light and heavy, dull
and sharp, subtle and gross, slimy and
rough, unmoving and mobile, turbid and
transparent, and solid and liquid.

These properties can be related to matter, thoughts, and ideas, and they are also related to the doshas. Particular substances that are characterized by specific gunas can increase or decrease dosha influence throughout the body.

An Ayurvedic practitioner takes into consideration all the qualities of the herbs themselves before prescribing treatment. For example, a vata-strengthening herb would be pungent, sour, or salty in its taste, or rasa. In addition, its characteristics, or gunas, might be light, dry, and cold, which would make it suitable for this type of dosha imbalance.

Herbs for the Doshas

Some of the best herbs for vata types include gotu kola and ginseng. Herbs for pitta types include aloe vera, comfrey, and saffron. Kapha types will respond well to elecampane and honey, which is used therapeutically in Ayurveda. (See also pages 166–71.)

AYURVEDIC HERBS

Herbs have been central to Ayurvedic practice for thousands of years. They are always prescribed in combination with advice about diet, exercise, and general lifestyle. Their rasas, or tastes, produce energies which promote their effects and encourage dosha balance. Many of the most commonly used Ayurvedic herbs are available and used in the West, including aloe vera, caraway, black pepper, and cinnamon. The boxes below and opposite show the characteristics and main uses of these useful herbs.

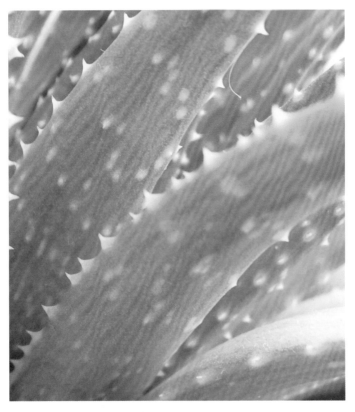

Aloe Vera

Properties: antiseptic, bitter, antiviral, cooling, and sweet. An astringent, and excellent blood cleanser, aloe vera calms all three doshas, and specifically reduces pitta (cools pitta rashes and ulcers).

Parts of plant used: leaf, gel, juice.

Conditions treated: thyroid, pituitary, and ovarian problems. Calms inflammation, soothes muscle spasm, purifies the blood, and cleanses the liver. Apply directly to the skin to heal burns, scalds, scrapes, sunburn, and wounds.

Cure-all
The aloe vera plant is often used in Ayurvedic medicine, and calms all three doshas.

Black Pepper

Properties: heating and drying. The taste is pungent and bitter, good for balancing an overabundance of kapha.

Parts of plant used: pepper kernel and oil.

Conditions treated: stimulates the plasma and the blood, the nervous system, the spleen, and the circulatory system, reduces fat, treats chronic indigestion, toxins in the colon, and sinus congestion.

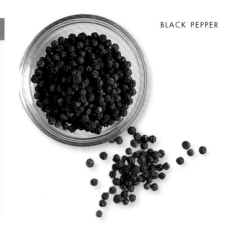

BLACK PEPPER

Caraway

Properties: antiseptic, antiviral, warming. A pungent, heating/drying agent, known for its stimulant properties.

Parts of plant used: seed.

Conditions treated: calms indigestion, reduces colic, flatulence, and accumulation of toxins and fluids. Reduces vata and kapha, and increases pitta. Clears kapha mucus build-up and soothes vata emotion, the muscles used in digestion, and menstrual cramps.

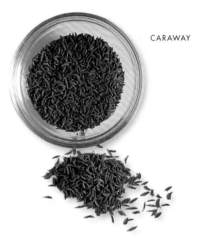

CARAWAY

Cinnamon

Properties: antiseptic, warming, pungent, sweet astringent, with stimulating, heating qualities. Acts as an anti-spasmodic, aphrodisiac, analgesic, and diuretic. Anti-bacterial, antifungal, used to treat gum disease, candida, and other yeast infections.

Parts of plant used: bark and leaf.

Conditions treated: dyspepsia, respiratory ailments, intestinal infections, scabies, and lice.

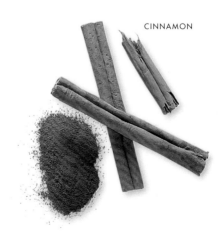

CINNAMON

Using Ayurvedic Herbs

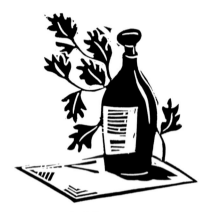

Herbal forms
There are a variety of different forms in which herbs can be prescribed in Ayurveda.

Many herbs used in Ayurvedic preparations are sold as pills, essences, powders, pastes, and concentrated remedies. Herbal remedies should be taken fresh because they will lose potency over time, unlike mineral remedies, which become stronger.

Herbal forms

The most common type of internal remedy prescribed in Ayurvedic medicine is tinctures. They are made by soaking the flowers, leaves, or roots of the herbs in alcohol in order to extract and preserve their properties.

Infusions & decoctions

With infusions, herbs are made into a "tea" using one teaspoon of dried herbs to one cup of boiling water. They are left to steep for 10 to 15 minutes, then strained, and drunk. Infusions are less concentrated than tinctures and are an easy way to take herbs at home. Similar to infusions, decoctions are made from tough materials, such as roots, barks, nuts, and seeds. Using the same proportions as for herbal tea, place the herb and water in a pan, bring to a boil, then simmer for 10 minutes. Strain and drink.

Suppositories & douches

Suppositories are ready-made for you to insert. Douches are made from an infusion or decoction that has been allowed to cool.

Oils

There are many Ayurvedic oils, prepared from plants, that are used in various ways, including massage and enemas.

Tablets & creams

Ayurvedic tablets and capsules are taken in the same way as prescription drugs. Ointments and creams are applied externally; the active ingredients pass through the pores of the skin into the blood stream.

Multi-herb Preparations

Herbal combinations are used to treat a variety of common problems.

- *Tiphala choornam* is one of the most popular Ayurvedic medicines for constipation and balancing the three doshas.

- *Yograj guggul* is very effective in rheumatism and osteoarthritis.

- *Avipatikar choornam* is useful for heartburn and for pacifying pitta.

- *Kanchar guggul* is used to cure lympadenitis and goiter.

- *Phal ghrit* is used widely as a cure for male and female infertility.

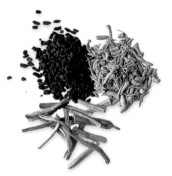

Vital herbs
The correct use of herbs and spices will rejuvenate your mind, body, and spirit.

REGENERATION
Following purification, regeneration is necessary to restore and stabilize the doshas. Regeneration, or rejuvenation (*rasayana* in Sanskrit), is intended to return your mind, body, and spirit to an earlier state of natural integration, to prevent diseases, and to minimize the effects of those diseases that cannot be avoided. The *Charaka Samhita* speaks of two types of rasayana, with substances and without.

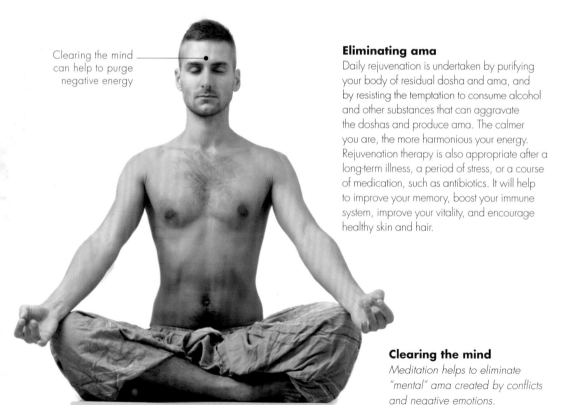

Clearing the mind can help to purge negative energy

Eliminating ama
Daily rejuvenation is undertaken by purifying your body of residual dosha and ama, and by resisting the temptation to consume alcohol and other substances that can aggravate the doshas and produce ama. The calmer you are, the more harmonious your energy. Rejuvenation therapy is also appropriate after a long-term illness, a period of stress, or a course of medication, such as antibiotics. It will help to improve your memory, boost your immune system, improve your vitality, and encourage healthy skin and hair.

Clearing the mind
Meditation helps to eliminate "mental" ama created by conflicts and negative emotions.

Herbal treatments

An Ayurvedic practitioner will use a variety of different herbs and other treatments for rejuvenation. Herbs that might be used include *ashwagandha* (winter cherry) for vata conditions, *shatavari* (*Asparagus racemosus*) for pitta conditions, and *pippali* (long pepper) for kapha conditions. Ashwagandha is bitter and astringent. It acts as a tonic, sedative, and aphrodisiac. It is prescribed for problems such as anxiety, insomnia, low libido, muscle weakness, chronic fatigue, and old age. Shatavari is used to help conditions such as diarrhea and dysentery, and kidney and liver problems, and as a tonic for the ovaries, endometrium, and fallopian tubes. All seven dhaatus are affected by its properties. Pippali is warming and sweet and can be used in the treatment of liver conditions, chronic dyspepsia, obesity, asthma, arthritis, and loss of appetite.

Drink of life

Many of the herbs suggested for rejuvenation can be drunk as teas.

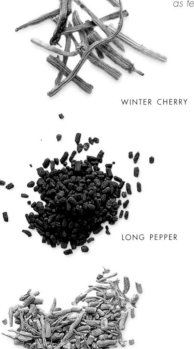

WINTER CHERRY

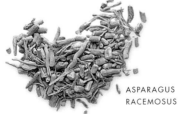

LONG PEPPER

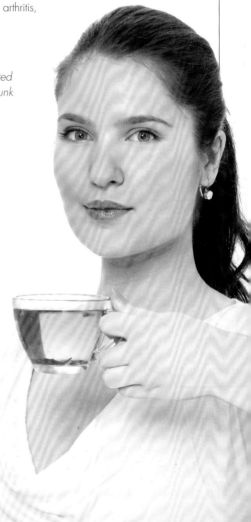

ASPARAGUS
RACEMOSUS

Regeneration Program

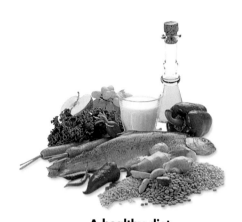

A healthy diet

Your nutritional status is one factor that Ayurvedic physicians use to decide the best treatment.

Rasayana, or rejuvenation therapy, forms one of the eight branches of Ayurveda. Regeneration is important in the ancient texts of Ayurveda, and a suitable rasayana agent will be selected by your practitioner, depending upon your age, individual constitution, adaptability, the condition of your sense organs, and your digestive capacity. Various rasayana medicines (normally herbs) are used to improve either your nutritional status or your digestive capacity and metabolic activity.

Prescriptions for health

Medhya rasayana are rasayana drugs used specifically to improve your intellect, memory, and willpower. *Naimittika rasayana* are drugs that are prescribed to improve your vitality when you have a specific disease.

There is also rejuvenation without medicines, called *acara rasayan*. Rejuvenating effects can be achieved when you practice good conduct, or *sadacara*. Sadacara includes finding time for spirituality; avoiding anger, jealousy, envy, and unkind behavior; avoiding the suppression of natural urges; and practicing meditation.

Sweetness in everything

One of the best ways to practice rasayana at home is to remember the keyword "sweetness." Think "sweet" thoughts, and be sweet in nature and in your approach to life. Your speech should promote harmony, your manner should be gently compassionate, your life routine simple, and your awareness calm and respectful of life and nature.

Healthy movement

Movement in the form of exercises or natural activities is important in Ayurveda and in regeneration, because it leaves you revitalized and helps you to work toward balance and harmony between mind and body. The tridosha exercises on the following pages are an important part of regeneration.

When to avoid exercise

According to Ayurveda, exercise is not good for very weak and emaciated people. It is also not appropriate after heavy meals or when you are feverish. Those with heart diseases, tuberculosis, asthma, or vertigo should not exercise. Vata people should have regulated exercise, preferably yoga, in moderation and should not engage in aerobic exercise.

On Aging

Ayurvedic rejuvenation helps your body and mind to retain their vigor in order that they will not interfere with your spiritual development as you grow older.

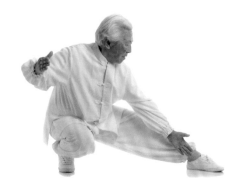

Gentle exercise

*T'ai chi is good exercise for
vata types, and all doshas
benefit from gentle stretching.*

EXERCISE FOR THE TRIDOSHAS Tridosha exercises are not just
important for regeneration (see pages 102–5). They also help to keep the balance
between vata, pitta, and kapha. Yoga is one of the most important types of exercise
for the mind and body, but there are other types of exercise that can be used to
balance the doshas.

Appropriate Exercise for Different Constitutions		
Vata	Pitta	Kapha
• yoga	• yoga	• yoga
• dancing (such as ballet)	• skiing	• tennis
• walking	• walking/jogging	• soccer
• hiking	• sailing/swimming	• running
• t'ai chi	• horseriding	• aerobics
• cycling	• hiking/mountaineering	• rowing

Active rest

*Relaxation and breathing are
vital parts of yoga practice,
which benefits all the doshas.*

Keeping active

Running is most suitable for kapha types, while a slow jog is appropriate for pittas.

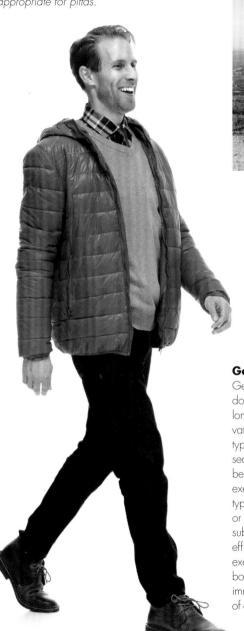

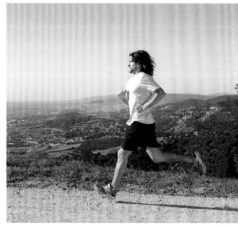

General principles

Gentle daily exercise is suggested for all three doshas. Only kapha types need a vigorous and long daily workout. Everyone else (and in particular vata types) needs only moderate exercise. Pitta types should exercise in moderation, avoiding hot seasons and midday sessions. Overexercising can be dangerous for vata types. If you choose strenuous exercise, make sure that you supplement it with some type of energy work, such as hatha yoga, t'ai chi, or qi gong. Energy work encourages all five of vata's subdoshas to remain within their spheres, cooperating efficiently with one another. Properly practiced, such exercise will stimulate the free flow of prana in your body, and encourage the development of better immunity and resilience by enhancing your production of ojas, or vital energy (see pages 62–63).

Yoga

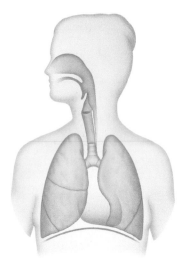

Breathing for life
Yoga encourages deep breathing and the free flow of prana through the body.

Yoga is one of the most important types of tridoshic exercise, and regular practice will encourage vitality and balance. The word *yoga* means "unity" or "oneness," and is derived from the Sanskrit word *yug*, which means "to join." In spiritual terms it refers to the union of the individual consciousness with the universal consciousness. On a practical level, yoga is a means of harmonizing the body, mind, and emotions, and is a tool that allows us to find a quiet space within. It utilizes the innate life force within the body and teaches us how to tap into, harness, and direct it skillfully. To achieve this, yoga uses movement, breath, posture, relaxation, and meditation, helping us to establish a healthy, balanced approach to living.

Types of posture

Yoga exercises consist of *asanas*, or postures, that involve stretching, bending, turning, and relaxing. Each posture has a specific therapeutic effect. There are six main groups of yoga postures: standing, inverted, twisting, back bend, forward bend, and side bend.

• Standing postures improve efficiency of the muscular, circulatory, respiratory, digestive, reproductive, endocrine, and nervous systems.

• Inverted postures balance the endocrine system and metabolism, enhance thinking power, and revitalize the internal organs.

• Twisting postures aid digestion, ease back pain, and improve intercostal (muscles between the ribs) breathing.

• Back bends are invigorating and encourage deep breathing.

• Forward bends improve the blood circulation, aid digestion, and calm troubled emotions.

• Side bends stimulate the body's main organs, such as the liver, kidneys, stomach, and spleen.

The relaxation and breathing exercises contained in the yoga tradition are important, and are designed to increase alertness and to let the previous exercises take effect. The best time to practice yoga is first thing in the morning or late in the afternoon. Each sequence should take between 10 and 15 minutes. You should never hold your breath while you are practicing yoga.

Breathe & Relax

When performing yoga positions, concentrate on your breath, clear your mind, and stop if it becomes painful or difficult to carry on.

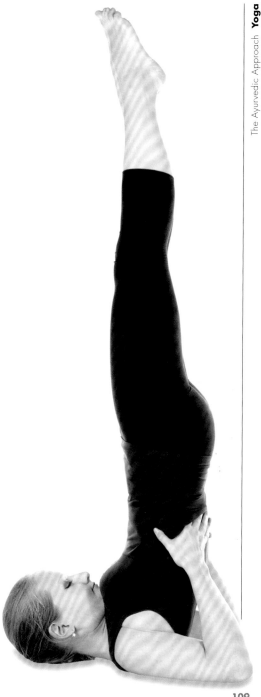

SALUTE TO THE SUN

One of the best yoga exercises to try at home is the Salute to the Sun (*surya namaskar*), which is a beautiful series of movements to loosen and energize the entire body. Practice it first thing in the morning as part of your daily routine. Perform the following sequence twice, relaxing after each completed sequence.

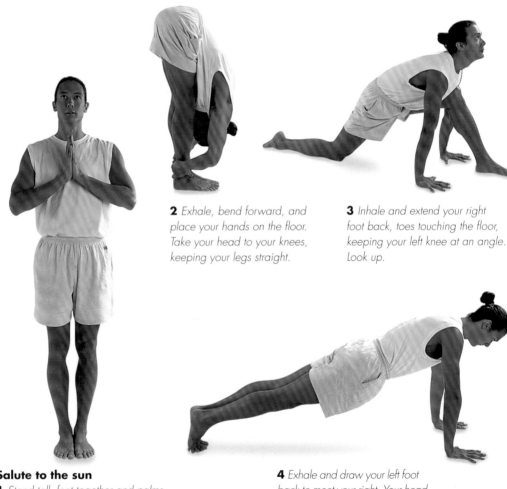

2 *Exhale, bend forward, and place your hands on the floor. Take your head to your knees, keeping your legs straight.*

3 *Inhale and extend your right foot back, toes touching the floor, keeping your left knee at an angle. Look up.*

Salute to the sun
1 *Stand tall, feet together and palms touching in front of the chest. Inhale and stretch your arms up and back.*

4 *Exhale and draw your left foot back to meet your right. Your head, back, and legs should form a straight line.*

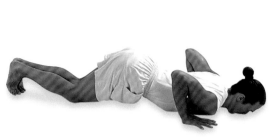

5 *Bend your arms and knees so your toes, knees, chest, hands, and forehead touch the floor.*

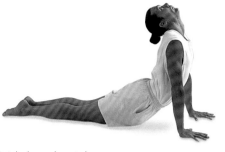

6 *Inhale and straighten your arms as you bend backward with your legs on the floor.*

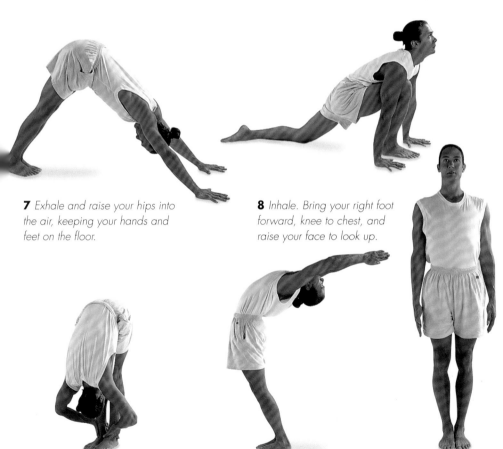

7 *Exhale and raise your hips into the air, keeping your hands and feet on the floor.*

8 *Inhale. Bring your right foot forward, knee to chest, and raise your face to look up.*

9 *Exhale. Draw your left foot to your right, your head to your knees, and straighten your legs.*

10 *Inhale. Come to standing, raise your arms over your head, and bend backward.*

11 *Exhale, stand up straight, and bring your hands to your sides.*

Yoga Exercises

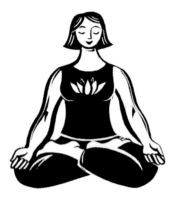

Uniting & integrating

The ultimate aim of yoga is to unite the individual soul with the universal, eternal spirit.

Yoga postures are designed to do much more than increase the flexibility of the physical body. The postures help to release and move stagnant energies and impurities that have accumulated in the marma points and the chakras. Asanas promote the unimpeded flow of energy through the mind and the body, and allow kundalini energy to travel up through the chakras. Yoga exercises should be done on an empty stomach and performed on the floor. Remove your glasses, contact lenses, and jewelry, and wear light, unrestricting clothing.

Releasing energy blocks

Before you begin it is important to remove accumulated tension from all parts of your body. The following movements will gently stretch your muscles, loosen the joints, and encourage deeper breathing. Hold each movement for a count of three and gradually increase the length of time as you progress.

Standing stretch

Stand tall, with your feet together. Inhale, raise your arms from your sides, and extend above head. Stretch, raising onto your toes, and hold. Exhale, lowering your arms to your sides. Repeat this procedure twice.

Side stretch

Stand tall, with your arms by your sides. Separate your feet so they are shoulders' width apart. Inhale, raise your right arm from the side, and extend above the head with the palm facing toward the left. Exhale and bend to the left.

Twist

Stand tall, with your feet a yard apart. Inhale, raise your arms in front to shoulder height. Exhale, rotate the arms to your right. Draw the left hand toward your right shoulder. Focus on your right hand as you turn from the waist as far as is comfortable, then hold. Inhale in this position. Exhale and return to front. Repeat on the opposite side, then lower your arms to the sides and relax.

Squat

Stand tall, with your feet hips' width apart. Raise your arms in front of you to shoulder height. Bend your knees and lower into a squat, trying to keep your heels on the ground.

Asanas

The word *asana* means "seating oneself in a comfortable position." Physical and mental relaxation are enhanced by yoga.

YOGA EXERCISES

The following asanas will encourage a harmonizing of the body, mind, and spirit. Whatever you do with the left side of your body must then be repeated with the right, to ensure balanced stretching. Ask a yoga instructor/or Ayurvedic practitioner for postures that are suitable for your constitutional type.

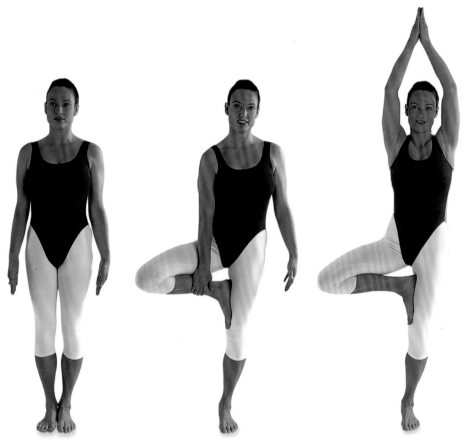

The Tree

1 *Stand tall, with your ankles touching and hands held by your sides. Relax the shoulders and look straight ahead.*

2 *Tuck the heel of your right foot into the inside of the left thigh, with your toes pointing downward and the right knee pointing out to the side.*

3 *Extend your arms above your head, bringing your palms together. Hold the pose for 30 seconds, then release.*

The Cobra

1 *Lie on your front, with legs straight and toes pointed. Place your chin on the floor.*

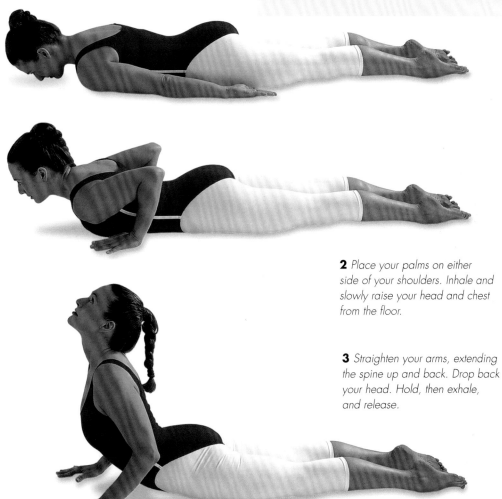

2 *Place your palms on either side of your shoulders. Inhale and slowly raise your head and chest from the floor.*

3 *Straighten your arms, extending the spine up and back. Drop back your head. Hold, then exhale, and release.*

115

Yoga Exercises

Most of the following postures, or asanas, are common and will be incorporated into most general yoga classes. If you are in any doubt about a posture, ask for help and a demonstration. Most of us will benefit from a weekly yoga class, in order to learn the techniques from an expert. They can then be practiced wherever you are and whenever you like.

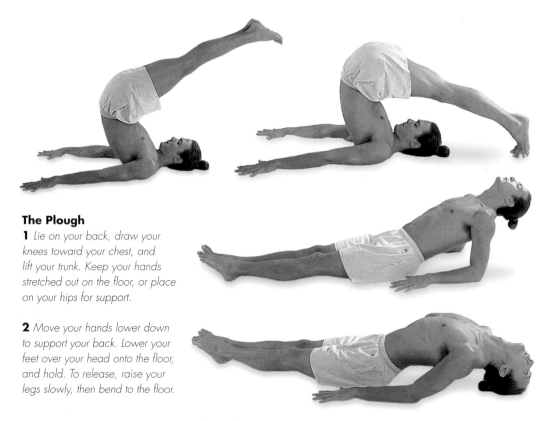

The Plough

1 Lie on your back, draw your knees toward your chest, and lift your trunk. Keep your hands stretched out on the floor, or place on your hips for support.

2 Move your hands lower down to support your back. Lower your feet over your head onto the floor, and hold. To release, raise your legs slowly, then bend to the floor.

The Fish

1 Lie down on your back. Place your elbows close to the side of your rib cage. Your arms should be flat on the floor.

2 Lean onto the elbows. Lift your head and place your crown gently on the floor. Draw the shoulder blades together, then hold, then release.

Safety first

When practicing the plough and the shoulder stand, place two folded blankets on the floor. Lie with your shoulders and arms on the blankets and head on the floor. This raises the torso above the head, easing pressure on the neck. Don't move your head when you are in, or moving in or out of, the poses. Check first with a doctor if you have any neck or back problems.

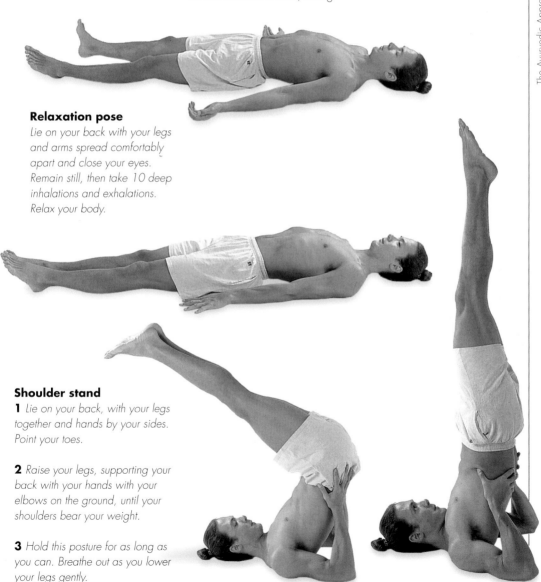

Relaxation pose

Lie on your back with your legs and arms spread comfortably apart and close your eyes. Remain still, then take 10 deep inhalations and exhalations. Relax your body.

Shoulder stand

1 *Lie on your back, with your legs together and hands by your sides. Point your toes.*

2 *Raise your legs, supporting your back with your hands with your elbows on the ground, until your shoulders bear your weight.*

3 *Hold this posture for as long as you can. Breathe out as you lower your legs gently.*

PRANAYAMA

PRANAYAMA An important part of both yoga and Ayurvedic philosophy is "right" breathing, which is known as *pranayama*. *Pranayama* is a Sanskrit word and can be defined as the science of breathing: *prana* means "life force" and *yama* means "control." Good health is possible only when we breathe fully and freely. We need plenty of oxygen in order to purify our blood and to burn up waste matter, and shortness or shallowness of breath often denotes anxiety or emotional unease.

The need for oxygen

Over the centuries, we have lost the art of breathing correctly. Most of us use only a tenth of our lung capacity, and in our busy, stressful lives this is becoming increasingly dangerous. When we do not have adequate oxygen, we suffer from fatigue, poor concentration, headaches, and various other conditions.

Controlling the life force

In Ayurveda, prana is the life force, and it is the power and energy behind breath. When we learn to control breathing, we can access the great reservoir of vital energy. We can create a proper rhythm of slow deep breathing, and these rhythmical patterns strengthen the respiratory system, soothe the nervous system, reduce craving and desire, free the mind, and improve concentration.

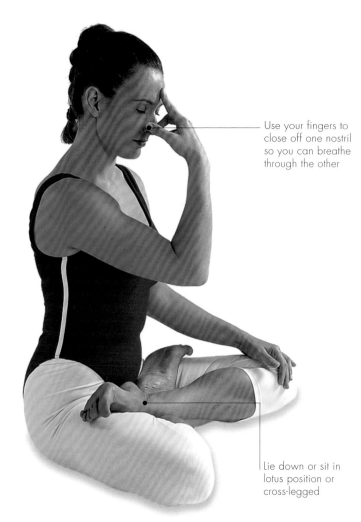

Use your fingers to close off one nostril so you can breathe through the other

Lie down or sit in lotus position or cross-legged

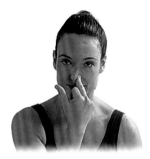

Kapha breathing
Kaphas should close the left nostril and breathe in through the right, release, and breathe out through the left.

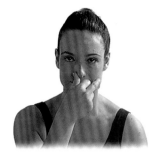

Pitta breathing
Pittas should repeatedly breathe in through the left nostril and breathe out through the right.

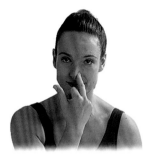

Vata breathing
Vatas benefit from alternate nostril breathing. Block one nostril and breathe in through the other; then change over and breathe out. Next, inhale through the nostril from which you just exhaled and so on.

Balancing the doshas
Recent research indicates that yogic breathing can successfully relieve conditions such as asthma, eczema, high blood pressure, and diabetes. Pranayama exercises can be prescribed according to your pre-dominant dosha, in order to help balance the three doshas in your mind and body.

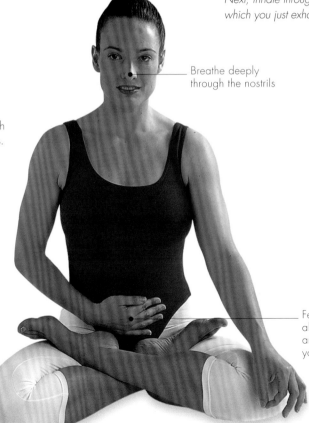

Breathe deeply through the nostrils

Feel your abdomen rise and fall with your breath

Pranayama Exercises

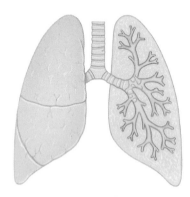

Using your lungs
Most of us use only a tenth of our lung capacity. Breathing correctly helps prevent illnesses and enhances well-being.

Ayurveda teaches that the pranayama breathing technique reconciles the opposite sides of our nature. The right nostril is connected to our active, rational side, while the left nostril is a link with our passive emotional side. Through alternate nostril breathing, we can bring the two sides into harmony. Ideally, pranayama exercises should be carried out while you are lying on your back or sitting down, although they can be done anywhere. Make sure you keep your head and back in alignment. Practice the exercises for five minutes every morning and evening.

As you practice the exercises, count slowly to yourself until you have mastered the art of breathing in a relaxed way.

Vitality breath

Take a deep breath in through both nostrils. To exhale, pull in your abdominal muscles and diaphragm in a sharp stroke that forces the air out of your nose so quickly that the breath is almost a sneeze.

As soon as you have exhaled, relax, then allow the breath to inhale naturally in a short burst. Exhalation should take less time than inhalation.

To begin with, perform the above vitality breath ten times at a rate of two exhalations per second.

This completes one cycle. Take a minute's rest between ending one cycle and beginning the next. Begin by completing two cycles and gradually build yourself up to five.

Bhastika breath

Breathe in and out three times. Inhale to fill your lungs to about a third of their capacity, then exhale. Repeat for ten breaths, using your lungs and rib cage as though they were bellows. Finally, inhale to fill your lungs as much as possible and then exhale.

Complete breath

Breathe in deeply from your abdomen, which will expand to the rib cage and up to your collarbone. Breathe out, feeling yourself deflate in reverse order to the inhalation.

Give your abdomen a gentle push to help to clear the breath from the bottom of your lungs. Breathe in deeply to a (slow) count of four, and then out, again to a count of four. As you become more practiced at the exercise, gradually increase to a count of eight.

Pranayama for Health

When it is practiced correctly, pranayama can reduce the incidence of asthma, bronchitis, sinus problems, and colds.

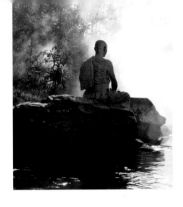

A powerful practice
Through deep meditation, we can reach a state of perfect harmony and enlightenment.

MEDITATION

In Ayurveda, meditation is an important way to stabilize the doshas and enhance well-being. Just as panchakarma cleanses the body, meditation cleanses the spirit. Western medicine has been slow to realize the benefits of meditation, but research has shown that it can slow your heart rate, reduce negative emotions, and produce a sense of calm. When we meditate, the kundalini energy can travel upward through the chakras and revitalize the organs (see page 90–93).

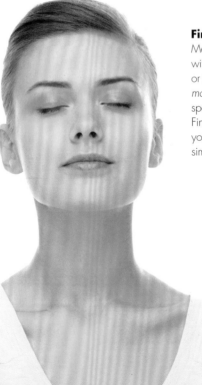

Find the peace within
Meditation is a tool to make us aware of the peace within us, a place that the outside world cannot touch or influence. The word meditation comes from the Latin *moderi*, meaning "to heal." Find a clean, naturally lit space and make an oasis of calm in which to meditate. Find a moment when your day is less fraught. When you feel calm and relaxed, and are sitting comfortably, simply allow your thoughts to flow.

A peaceful space
Sit comfortably and breathe deeply and rhythmically. The everyday world feels far away.

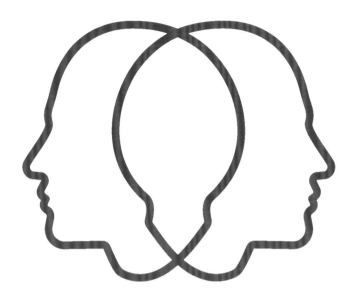

Quieting the thoughts

Emptying the mind is an artificial act. Thoughts must continue on their natural path until they reach the silent place. Imagine yourself exploring the rooms of your mind, washing each one clean with a burst of radiant white light. Let thoughts enter your head, and then let them recede on the waves of light. Let your thoughts progress from room to room. Each chamber of the mind can offer you insight.

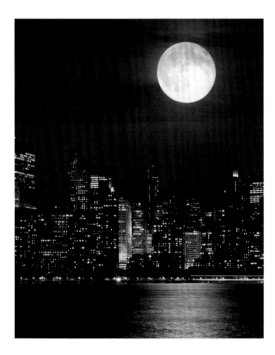

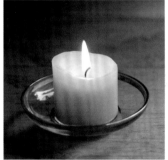

Let the light in

Use a flickering candle—the eternal flame—to guide you along the meditative path.

Lunar energy

Meditate in the quiet, cool dark of a moonlit room to find the light within yourself.

The Importance of Meditation

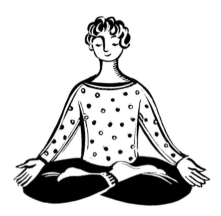

Spiritual peace
Meditation forms an essential part of Ayurveda, and helps to promote holistic well-being.

The yogi Amrit Desai once said, "Prayer is you talking to God. Meditation is you listening to God." Meditation puts you in touch with the spiritual side of yourself, which can have a dramatic effect on your physical and emotional well-being.

According to research undertaken in fifty countries around the world, meditation improves intelligence, increases creativity, improves perception, improves orderliness, lowers blood pressure, reduces anxiety, reduces your requirement for medical care, decreases stress, reverses the aging process, changes your breathing, promotes deep relaxation, increases productivity, improves your mood, and increases your self-awareness and self-esteem.

As part of an Ayurvedic lifestyle, it will help to improve your health on all levels—bringing spirit into the mind-body equation.

Deep rest

Meditation provides the mind and body with a unique and profound state of restful alertness. The body gains an extraordinarily deep state of rest while the mind settles down to a state of inner calm and wakefulness.

This process dissolves deeply rooted stress and tension, rejuvenates the entire system, infuses the mind with creativity and intelligence, and provides the basis for dynamic, successful activity. How this works is largely unknown. In Ayurveda it is believed that meditation works on the chakras (see pages 92–93), encouraging the flow of prana upward, to embody and expand spirit.

Stress relief

Meditation has a uniquely relaxing effect on the body, and it is a scientifically validated technique for providing your entire system with very deep—profound—rest. This profound rest has been shown to release accumulated stress and tension that no other form of relaxation—including a restful vacation, relaxation exercises, physical exercise, or anything else—has come close to eliminating.

The End of the Day

Try to meditate for 20 to 30 minutes at the end of your day to calm your mind and encourage restful sleep. Regenerative energy will move more efficiently while you sleep.

A SIMPLE MEDITATION EXERCISE

Meditation should ideally be learned from an experienced instructor, but you can practice it at home—alone or in a group. Always try to meditate at the same time each day and in the same place if possible. Begin with five minutes or so of deep breathing, and then breathe a little more gently, with a regular rhythm from the abdomen.

Preparation

Sit cross-legged on the floor with your hands outstretched and your palms facing upward. You can meditate with your eyes opened or closed, whichever feels best to you. Many people find it helpful to have a mantra, which is a syllable, a word, or a phrase that you repeat to yourself (aloud or silently) as a chant (see pages 128–29).

What to do

The idea of meditation is to purify the mind and let your own natural energy flow within you. There is no wrong way to meditate. Try this simple exercise to begin.

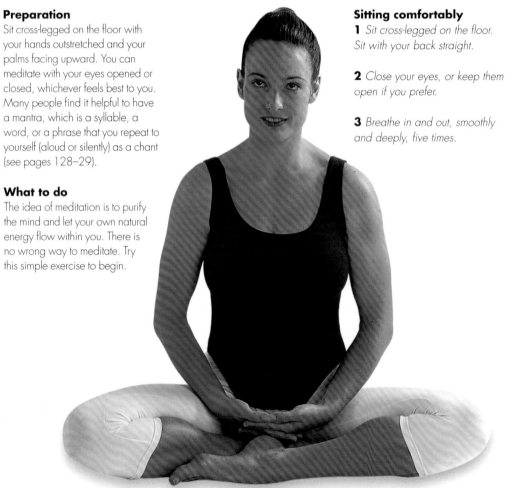

Sitting comfortably

1 *Sit cross-legged on the floor. Sit with your back straight.*

2 *Close your eyes, or keep them open if you prefer.*

3 *Breathe in and out, smoothly and deeply, five times.*

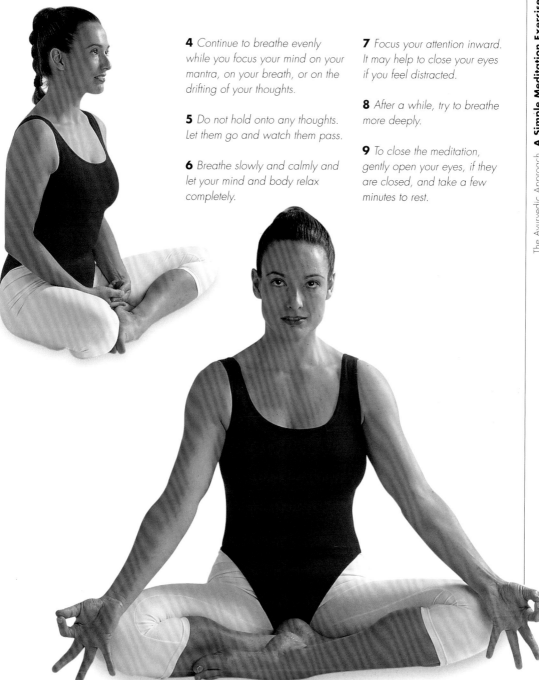

4 Continue to breathe evenly while you focus your mind on your mantra, on your breath, or on the drifting of your thoughts.

5 Do not hold onto any thoughts. Let them go and watch them pass.

6 Breathe slowly and calmly and let your mind and body relax completely.

7 Focus your attention inward. It may help to close your eyes if you feel distracted.

8 After a while, try to breathe more deeply.

9 To close the meditation, gently open your eyes, if they are closed, and take a few minutes to rest.

Mantras

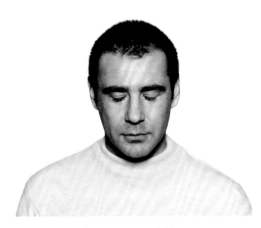

The power within

*Mantras can help to heal
those illnesses caused by
negative karma.*

Types of healing

According to Ayurveda, there are three categories of healing:

• The highest type of healing is spiritual (sattvic) and undertaken purely by prayer and mantra.

• The second type is human (rajasic) and is undertaken with medicine and purification therapies.

• The third and lowest type of healing is tamasic, where healing is by surgery.

Spiritual power

All mantras are directed toward specific deities, and in Ayurveda prominent healing deities include Vishnu or Dhanwantari (the god of Ayurveda), Shiva, Krishna, and Durga. Powerful Ayurvedic herbs also have specific deities that are said to rule them.

Mantras range from those that will cure a patient of the illness that they are suffering from, to those that will enable the patient to live a healthy and prosperous life. There are also mantras that will help you to liberate yourself from the endless cycle of birth and rebirth, and attain *moksha* (liberation).

Mantras that provide spiritual healing are an important part of Ayurveda. These have been neglected recently, due in part to the colonial period in India and to the influence of Western education in India. Mantras are clearly prescribed in the ancient texts of Ayurveda, and it has been acknowledged by spiritually inclined Ayurvedic doctors that mantras and ritual can play an important—if not the most vital role— in curing all but very minor ailments.

Using mantras

Mantras can be *bija* mantras, with single or "seed" syllables making simple sounds, or they can be rhythmic chants called *mala* mantras. All mantras can be enunciated in your mind or chanted aloud, but the former is more effective for healing body ailments and for spiritual progress.

Because using mantras is a practice that can help in the process toward spiritual awakening, Ayurveda believes that only a true spiritual master can guide you in their use. In Ayurveda, the practice of mantras involves knowing the name of the original seer of the mantra, its secret seed syllable, and the key to its use, and an armour *kavach*. Using a mantra without also incorporating these codes is said to be ineffective and sometimes even dangerous.

Spiritual Gift

Mantras form an intricate system of meditation. Only a spiritually trained Ayurvedic doctor or a true guru can instruct you properly in the science and use of a mantra.

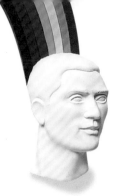

Expanded consciousness
Using the senses to their fullest extent helps you to experience the world more colorfully.

TRAINING YOUR SENSES
One of the mandates of Ayurveda is that we make full use of our senses, in order fully to experience the world and, through that, nature, healing, and good health. Our sensory impressions can influence the workings of the mind and the emotions. Smells, colors, sounds, objects that we touch, and everything that we taste can influence our state of balance and harmony. When the doshas are disturbed, using our senses can help to bring them back into alignment.

Healing senses
Many of the therapies in Ayurveda involve using the senses to heal. For example, Ayurvedic herbalism groups herbs and foods according to their tastes, while mantras use the repetition of sound for spiritual healing. Aromatic oils that stimulate the areas of the brain responsible for emotion are used in various therapies, including massage, which can also enhance your sense of touch.

Dosha strengths
The senses of the different doshas develop to different degrees. Vata is characterized by good hearing and taste.

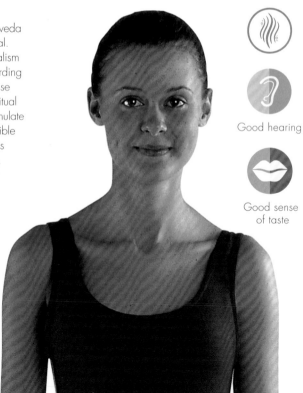

Good hearing

Good sense of taste

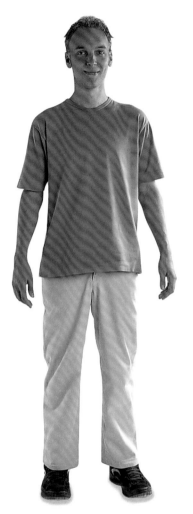

Strong visual
perception

Good sense
of taste

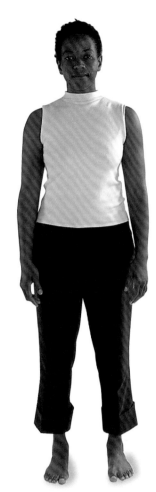

Good sense
of smell

Good sense
of taste

Achieving harmony

The five senses correspond to the five elements. Sound is transmitted through ether; air, which Ayurveda teaches is related to the nervous system, is believed to correspond to touch; fire relates to sight; water is necessary for taste; and earth is connected with the sense of smell. When all of the senses are balanced (used appropriately),

we are more in tune with the world around us and more likely to achieve harmony. In Ayurveda, training the senses involves using each of them equally. For example, if we fail to use our sense of taste properly by eating bland, unwholesome foods, and have too many baths and massages, we will enter into a state of imbalance. The idea is to use all senses equally and to educate them.

Pitta & kapha

A pitta type, left, may have excellent visual faculties, while a kapha, right, may have a strong sense of taste and smell.

In Tune with Nature

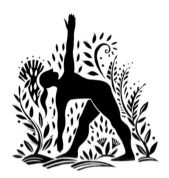

Natural causes
*The natural world can have
a dramatic impact on our health
and well-being.*

According to Ayurvedic philosophy, humans are arranged in exactly the same way as the universe or the world around them. In other words, the microcosm (human life) is an exact replica of the macrocosm (universe). For this reason, our health (on all levels) is inextricably linked to the universe and the rhythms of nature. Ayurvedic practitioners believe that if we allow ourselves to be guided by the natural world around us, we can regulate the balance of our inner energies naturally. The rhythm of waxing and waning in the world around us is central to our own minds and bodies. Plants and animals, who have no real sense of time, use nature to keep them in sync with the seasons. If we wish to live healthily, we need to synchronize ourselves actively with nature's rhythms. Ayurveda recognizes four main "seasonal" cycles that apply to men and women alike. Establishing a rhythm in each of these cycles is essential for physical health, and it helps you to flow in the most appropriate direction for you and your dosha type.

Chronobiology
This specialized branch of biology researches the relationship between life events and the natural laws of chronology. Researchers have discovered that there is a connection between the natural rhythm of the cosmos and the human biorhythms. If we learn to live in harmony with the rhythms of the day, the season, the year, and the stage that we have reached in our life cycle (see page 138–39), we will function more efficiently and experience a sense of well-being.

Day & night
From dawn to midmorning is kapha time, as the system is stimulated by wakefulness

and sunlight. From midmorning to midafternoon, pitta is most active. After this comes an increasing vata force, which is at its peak at dusk.

Kapha predominates from dusk through slightly more than the first third of the night, pitta rules the midnight hours, and vata accumulates through the pre-dawn hours. Over the course of 24 hours, pitta predominates during the day, vata rules over dawn and dusk, and kapha predominates at night.

Dosha Time

Using the doshas to guide you in eating, working, and exercising can improve the effectiveness and harmony of your day.

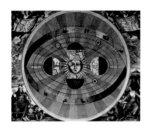

Natural cycle
Our physical bodies work in tandem with the movement of the earth around the sun.

THE AYURVEDIC TIME CLOCK
The influence of the doshas varies according to the time of day or night. Ayurveda divides the 24 hours into two principal cycles, which are in turn composed of three phases. Each of these phases is governed by one dosha.

Vata dominates between two and six o'clock in the early morning and in the afternoon, often the best times for physical or mental activity. However, it is important not to overwork or overexercise during these times.

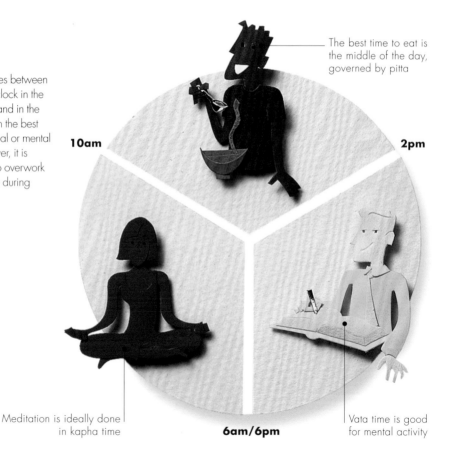

The best time to eat is the middle of the day, governed by pitta

10am

2pm

Meditation is ideally done in kapha time

6am/6pm

Vata time is good for mental activity

Pitta is most active in the middle of both day and night. We are at our strongest during the midday pitta phase, which is why you may feel very hungry then. Pitta is responsible for converting food into energy; therefore it is important to eat the main meal at lunchtime. At night, pitta uses its fire for keeping the body warm during sleep.

Kapha is most dominant in the early morning and evening. Kapha problems, such as excess mucus, sinusitis, and asthma, may become worse during these hours. Use kapha times (in the morning in particular) to purify your body and mind (through yoga, meditation, and detoxification therapies) and tend to your personal needs.

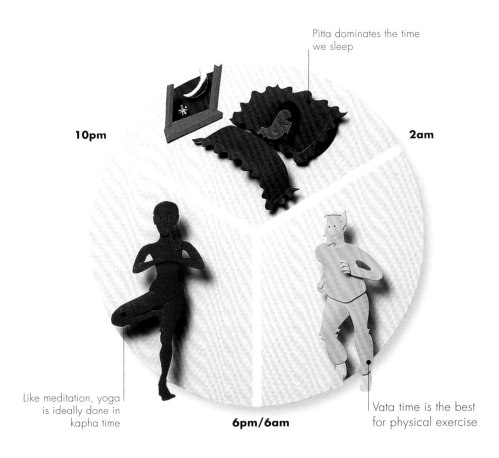

Pitta dominates the time we sleep

10pm

2am

Like meditation, yoga is ideally done in kapha time

6pm/6am

Vata time is the best for physical exercise

The Ayurvedic Seasons

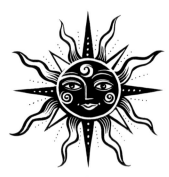

Ritucharya
Seasonal routines, called ritucharya, are important for strength, health, and energy.

Just as our bodies and minds are affected by the time of day, they are also influenced by the changing seasons. Part of this effect may be due to the fact that our bodies respond to different degrees of light and darkness, heat and cold, and damp, wet, and dryness. In India, there are six seasons: *Shishira* (winter), *Vasantha* (spring), *Greeshma* (summer), *Varsha* (rainy season), *Sarath* (fall), and *Hemantha* (the cold period before winter). In the West we have three seasons according to the Ayurvedic point of view: kapha season, from mid-March to mid-June; pitta season, from mid-June to mid-October; and vata season, mid-October to mid-March.

Living with the seasons

Ayurveda suggests that we prepare for each seasonal change by detoxifying the body and mind (see page 74). Pitta-related problems are most common at the beginning of its season, and vata-type problems tend to build up in the late fall. Kapha problems increase during the rainy season in India and are more common in the periods before winter and summer.

When in a season corresponding to your dosha type, you will need to take extra care during that period. Doshas are more likely to become unbalanced throughout these seasons. You will need to avoid long-term extremes of the type of temperature that is most dangerous for your constitutional type. For example, vata types will need to avoid excessive cold, wind, rain, or snow, and pitta types will need to avoid very hot or dry weather. Ayurveda also recommends that you adjust your diet to the seasons (see pages 162–63), according to your constitution.

In general, however, everyone must be aware of how seasonal changes affect the body, and take steps to change diet and lifestyle in order to put the least pressure on your body. In summer, for example, drinking cold water and cooking foods that do not aggravate pitta is useful. A high-protein and high-carbohydrate diet has a cooling effect, and you should avoid warm baths at this time. In winter, waste products can build up, causing energy blockages. This is the time to eat heating, warm, and cooked foods, as well as to drink warm water and other warming drinks. Warm clothing and baths are also recommended.

Seasons of the Doshas

In most countries, kapha dominates in spring, pitta takes over during the summer, and vata, climaxes in fall, then gradually becomes calmer over the winter as kapha rises.

THE RHYTHM OF LIFE

There is a third cycle that relates to and affects the three doshas in Ayurveda. Our lives are divided into the three stages of youth, middle age, and old age. Each stage has different characteristics which correspond to the doshas. During each dosha-predominant period, it is useful to adopt a diet, lifestyle, and therapeutic treatments that will balance a dosha that is in danger of becoming misaligned. Taking account of the dosha dominating your stage of life will, again, help you to establish harmony with the cycles of nature.

Family harmony

Understanding which doshas predominate at different stages of life can help to encourage health and harmony.

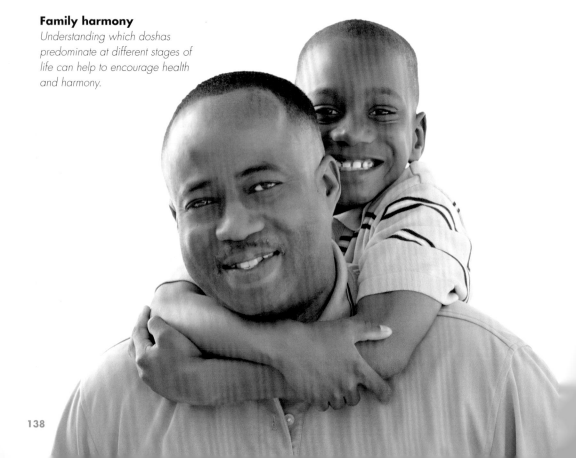

Early life

Childhood is considered to be a kapha time. From birth to about the age of 20 to 30, you can expect to experience more kapha-related problems, such as colds, coughs, and asthma. This is a stage of physical, emotional, and intellectual growth and development.

Active life

During the mid-life pitta phase, most people should aim to take regular exercise.

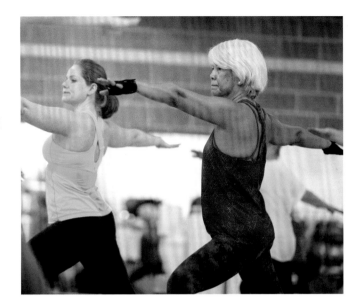

The middle years

Pitta dominates the phase between the years of 20 to 30 and 50 to 60. This is a period characterized by active, full, independent living. Pitta-related problems are more common at this time.

Later life

The last phase of our lives is, therefore, vata-dominated. Vata accelerates after age 50 or 60, as the mind, body, and spirit gradually disintegrate. Vata-type conditions, such as arthritis, memory loss, wrinkles, dry skin, and constipation may occur. During this period, our powers of recovery are diminished, and all of us will benefit from adopting a pure diet and reducing excess physical activity.

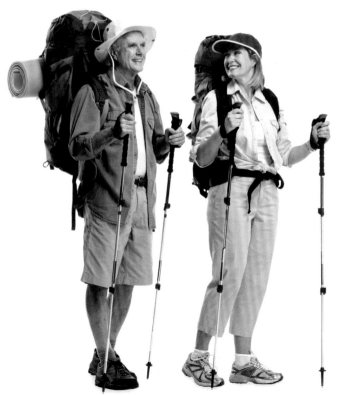

Daily Living with Ayurveda

The daily program for living in Ayurveda is called *dinachariya*. It offers guidelines that help us to achieve optimum well-being.

By following a lifestyle that is in harmony with the natural cycle of the day, and basing our daily activities around it, we reinforce our own innate strength and intelligence. Ayurveda recommends that you try to keep your days as close to the same routine as possible, every day of the year. This will also help to stabilize your emotions. It is important to achieve a harmonious rhythm in your day.

Morning

- Wake before sunrise if possible. The body functions best on an early start. Move slowly, and take time to plan your day.

- Evacuate your bladder and bowels. Drinking a glass of lukewarm water upon rising can help to encourage this.

- Clean your teeth, tongue, hands, and face. A clean tongue is essential for the sense of taste. Ayurvedic toothpastes and gargles are available from health-food stores.

- Sniff two drops of sesame seed oil into each nostril to encourage your sense of smell.

- Practice self-massage every day if you are a vata type, or less often if you are a kapha or pitta type (see pages 82–83).

- Take some form of physical exercise before eating breakfast. This will improve your circulation and stabilize your doshas. Yoga is an ideal exercise because it can be done at any time of year, in any place. Choose an exercise that is appropriate to your constitutional type (see pages 114–15).

- Bath or shower. Cleanliness is essential before beginning your day.

- Dress in clean, comfortable clothing, and find a space where you can meditate.

- Meditate for 10 to 20 minutes, longer if possible, depending on how much time you have in the morning before your activities of the day begin.

- Have a light breakfast before eight o'clock.

- Clean your teeth and your tongue after every mealtime.

- If possible, take a short walk after breakfast to encourage the digestive process.

Daytime

- Use the daylight hours to engage in your work or to study.

- Have a healthy lunch—this should be the main meal of your day. Choose foods that are appropriate both to the seasons and to your constitution. Do not eat too much—the right quantity of food is the amount that can be scooped up with two hands.

- Eat at a normal pace—not too slowly or too quickly—and try to eat in silence. Drinking with meals weakens digestion.

Evening

- At at time near to sunset, practice evening meditation for 10 to 20 minutes.

- Eat your evening meal early, in order for it to be properly digested before going to bed. It should be light and easily digestible. Once again, take a walk to encourage digestion.

- Engage in light and enjoyable activities during the evening.

- Go to bed before 10pm, so that you can fall asleep when kapha energy predominates and supports sleep. Between 10pm and 2am, pitta energy becomes more dominant and sleep may therefore be less restful.

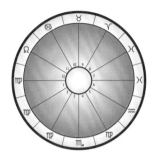

Cosmic clues

In India, it is common to consult a Vedic astrologer to assess whether the planets are to blame for chronic illnesses.

ASTROLOGY
This is a branch of Vedic philosophy that works together with Ayurvedic science. Practitioners often undertake predictive astrology (*jyotish*) to find out whether you have certain predilections for particular diseases at different times. The remedies for some of the astrological situations include gems and mantras. These two forms of treatment were part of Ayurvedic training in ancient times. Today, much of this knowledge has been diluted and lost. Astrology does not form part of Ayurvedic practice in the West, but all practitioners are aware of its importance.

Part of the cosmos

What happens on earth and in the heavens is directly related, and for thousands of years humans have known that astrological influences, signs, and portents cannot be ignored. In most areas of India, the exact time of birth is recorded so that the astrologer can produce a chart showing the planetary influences to be expected during a child's lifetime.

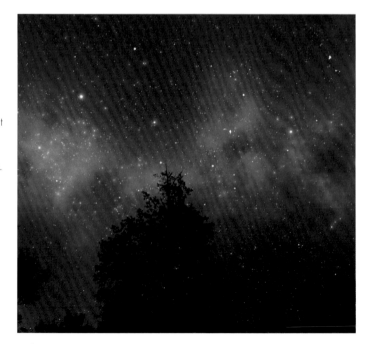

The sky reveals

According to Ayurveda, there is indisputable evidence that the planets influence disease.

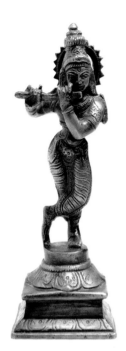

Religious icon
The planets, which can cause illnesses, are represented as deities in Hinduism.

Planetary influences
The position of the natal moon (the moon at birth) is important in deciding the prakrithi, or constitutional type, of the individual, and the movements of the moon provide a strong influence on human healing. According to Indian astrology, crises in acute diseases are marked by the transiting moon, and the most serious crisis in any acute disease occurs on the fourteenth day when the moon is in opposition to the day when the disease started. *Nakshatras* (lunar stars) are important influences on health and other aspects of life. Other planets in unfavorable positions can also affect health (see box). Rahu and ketu are lunar nodes, points in space where the moon crosses the path of the sun in the sky. Rahu is the ascending node and ketu is descending.

Planets	Diseases	Natural Aids
SUN	Diseases of the eye, blood, and nervous system, cancer, viral infections, and heart problems	Honey, saffron, cardamom
MOON	Mental illness, obesity, gynecological, urinary, and bacterial problems	Lotus, coral
MARS	Viral infections, eye, heart, and digestive problems	Sandalwood
MERCURY	Insomnia, neurosis, hypertension, and accidents	Gold dust
JUPITER	Diabetes, rheumatism, and arthritis	Pepper, sugar cane
VENUS	Sexual, gynecological, and kidney problems	Any spice
SATURN	Kidney problems, rheumatism, and arthritis	Shatavari (*Asparagus racemosus*)
RAHU	Accidents and surgical problems	Multanga (*Cyperus rotundus*)
KETU	Accidents and surgical problems	Brahmi (*Centella asiatica*)

The Moon's Influence

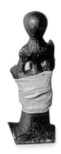

Divine planets

The worship of particular planets is part of spiritual healing in Ayurveda.

Astrology is the barometer of karma and reveals the influences that you are born under. Unlike in Western astrology, the position of the moon is very important in Vedic astrology. The 27 nakshatras (constellations of the moon or lunar stars) are the basis for analyzing and planning all of life's major events, from marriage to moving house, as well as deciding the vata, pitta, and

Pisces	Aries	Taurus	Gemini
part of Poorvabhadra part of Uttrabadhra Revati	Aswini Bharani part of Kartika	part of Kartika Rohini part of Mrgasirsa	part of Mrgasirsa Ardra part of Punarvasu
Cancer	**Leo**	**Virgo**	**Libra**
part of Punarvasu Pushya Asleshaw	Makha Pubba part of Uttra	part of Uttra Hasta part of Chitra	part of Chitra Swati part of Visakha
Scorpio	**Sagittarius**	**Capricorn**	**Aquarius**
part of Visakha Anuradha Jyeshta	Moola Poorvabhadra part of Uttrabadhra	part of Uttrabadhra Sravana part of Dhanista	part of Dhanista Stabisha part of Poorvabhadra

kapha constitution in individuals. They are even used to decide the best days for treatment—you should avoid starting treatment on a day when the lunar star is the same as your birth sign, for example, or during *chandrashtama* (see below). The lunar stars are listed in the box opposite, under the constellations in which they are sited.

Moon phases

The transit of the moon in the eighth house to your natal moon is called *chandrashtama*. This particular phase is characterized by two troublesome days when nothing seems to go right, and will occur at least once a month.

To calculate when the moon is in your eighth house, you need to know in which house, or sign, the moon was when you were born (your natal moon). You then count eight houses along. For example, if the moon was in the sign of Aries when you were born, whenever the moon transits the sign of Scorpio there will be difficult days for you.

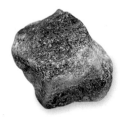

Lapis lazuli
This colorful stone can be used to help kaphas raise their energy to a more refined level.

GEM THERAPY
One of the best ways to address astrologically induced illness is through gem therapy. The power of different gems, which are associated with different illnesses (see box opposite), is taken particularly seriously by Vedic astrologers, who can determine which stones or crystals to use according to the circumstances of your life chart.

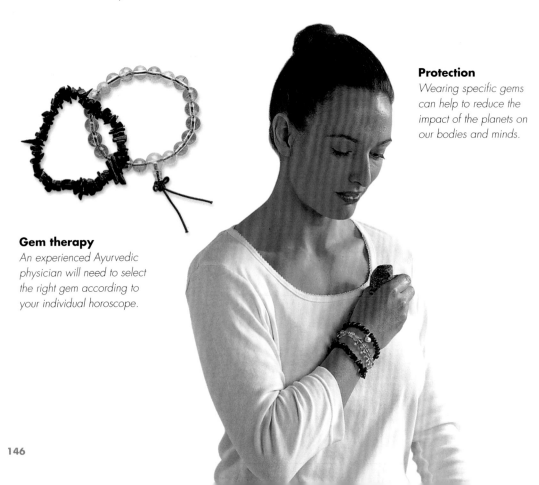

Protection
Wearing specific gems can help to reduce the impact of the planets on our bodies and minds.

Gem therapy
An experienced Ayurvedic physician will need to select the right gem according to your individual horoscope.

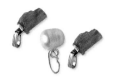

Jewelry to soothe
Wearing a gem next to your skin will help you to take in its healing energy.

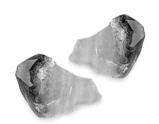

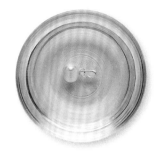

Vata stone
Amethyst stones are used in Ayurvedic medicine to help correct an imbalance of vata.

Healing drink
Water absorbs the properties of gems, so you can soak them overnight, then drink the water.

Common Illnesses	Associated Gems
Rheumatism and musculoskeletal problems	red coral, emerald, pearl, dark-blue sapphire, ruby
Digestive diseases and diabetes	red coral, white coral, emerald
Diseases of the nervous system	dark-blue sapphire
Psychological disorders, including hysteria	emerald at night, red coral during the day
Skin diseases	white coral, yellow sapphire
Urinary and gynecological problems	pearl, diamond, red coral, yellow sapphire, emerald, topaz
Dental problems	sapphire, red coral
Ear, nose, and throat problems	yellow sapphire, white coral
Blood-related problems, such as anemia	dark-blue sapphire, emerald, ruby

Using Gem Therapy

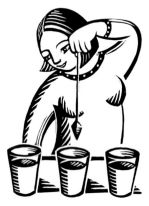

Choose carefully

*The wrong gem can aggravate
health conditions. The correct
stone can be used in the
treatment of disease.*

Although gem therapy is closely associated with astrology in Ayurveda, it can also be used without it. Gems and crystals have particular healing qualities and may be used in Ayurvedic medicine to treat certain diseases. Particular stones can also be used to reduce or increase the doshas. You can use gems and crystals on a day-to-day basis to affect your health and well-being. Try one of the following ways of using gems, depending on your dosha.

Vata

Topaz is a warm stone that was traditionally used to dispel fear, which is associated with vata. It calms anxiety. Wear topaz when you need to feel confident.

Amethyst is a good crystal to wear when you want to balance vata. It promotes clarity of mind and encourages harmony.

Pitta

Pearls and mother-of-pearl have the ability to reduce inflammatory conditions, and those affecting the emotions. Pearls are also used to treat rheumatism, bone diseases, and musculoskeletal problems. Natural pearls should be worn as a first choice, although cultured pearls are also effective. Begin wearing your pearls on a Monday (the moon's day) during a new moon. Don't wear pearls if you are suffering from a kapha-related condition, such as a cold. Moonstone is a good gem for reducing excess pitta since it calms emotions and is cooling.

Kapha

Excess kapha can be reduced using lapis lazuli, which helps kapha types to raise their bodily vibrations from dense and

slow to refined and resonating. Lapis
lazuli is known as the heavenly stone.
Ruby will also reduce excess kapha.
Wear it set in gold or silver to encourage
strength and resolve.

How to use gemstones

The atoms inside gemstones and crystals
are arranged in a very ordered pattern.
Create an essence containing the
energy pattern of a gemstone or crystal
by leaving the stone in a bowl of water
overnight. First make sure that the mineral
is not toxic, and that it does not dissolve
in water. The energized water can then
be drunk. The energies of gemstones can
also be transmitted when they are worn
next to the skin.

Gemstones & the Chakras

Gemstones are thought to affect the chakras:
for example, wearing a gemstone next to the
heart chakra will affect your emotional energy.

DIET & LIFESTYLE

According to Ayurveda, healthy living is a daily balancing act in which you care for yourself on every level: physical, emotional, and spiritual. Diet and lifestyle form the foundations of Ayurveda, and any other treatments suggested will be far less effective if you do not absorb and practice the principles. Ayurvedic medicine is founded on the belief that all disease stems from the digestive system, and the principles concentrate to a large extent on nutrition. Once you have learned how to eat and live in accordance with your dosha, you will begin to heal your vikruthi (or state of imbalance) and live in harmony.

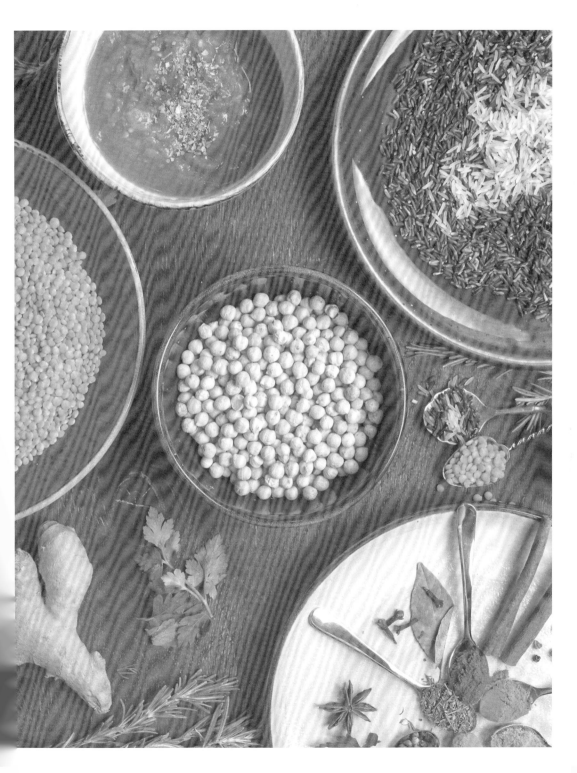

Simple Guidelines for Healthy Living

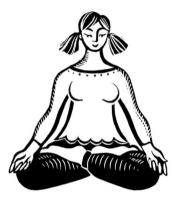

Quiet time
Making space in your life for meditation is an excellent way to calm the mind and spirit.

Ayurvedic practitioners believe that if people are cheerful, happy, and positive, they will improve their health and well-being. This belief has been echoed in recent Western research, which has shown that optimism can boost immunity and promote longevity. The following guidelines are recommendations for positive living to help you boost your health. They are suitable for most people, but an Ayurvedic practitioner may suggest alternatives

to these guidelines according to your presenting symptoms and dosha.

Eating calmly

Choose wholesome foods that look and taste good. Eat in a calm atmosphere and think about what you are eating. Try to eat at the same time each day; eat slowly, and chew thoroughly.

Never eat if you are not hungry, and always take some time to relax after meals. Take a walk if you can, to encourage good digestion.

Soothing the spirit

Do not suppress emotions or thoughts. If it is impossible to release them naturally, write them down or discuss them with a friend. Every day, find time to meditate, to unite the mind, body, and spirit.

Set aside some time to relax each day—use essential oils, if necessary, to calm an unbalanced dosha. Avoid sleeping on your back or your stomach, as energy centers respond better if you sleep on your side.

Incorporate self-massage (see pages 82–85) into your day, and follow it with a bath. Exercise according to the needs of your dosha (see pages 106–7). Most people need some form of daily exercise, such as yoga.

Conserving energy

Restrict your time on the computer and avoid lengthy intellectual activity, which provokes vata. Ayurveda recommends avoiding sex during menstruation, as it can cause vata imbalance. They also suggest avoiding masturbation and oral sex, which are considered a waste of energy.

Moral Principles

Live your life according to Ayurvedic principles: resist negative thoughts; abstain from verbal and physical abuse; do not give into greed or sorrow, do not hold onto anger; and avoid pride, arrogance, and ego.

AN AYURVEDIC DIET

Food is intended to supply energy (prana) to nourish the body and feed the mind, and a good diet will ensure that your weight is balanced and that you feel vital, physically strong, and healthy. Your diet should be chosen according to the seasons, your individual constitution, and any specific dosha imbalances that are present. According to Ayurvedic philosophy, our health and well-being depend upon how well our digestive system provides nutrition for the physical body. This is determined not only by the substances that we choose to eat, but also by the way that they are processed and assimilated.

Food types

Food is divided into two types: heavy and light. Heavy foods, which include potatoes, bread, and rice, are difficult to digest; while light foods, such as cooked vegetables and juices, are more easily digested. A properly balanced meal will consist of three parts heavy foods to one part light. In the evening, you may choose to eat more light food, to place less pressure on the digestive system.

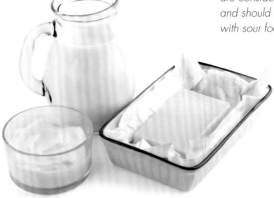

Dairy produce

Milk, butter, and cream are considered sweet, and should not be eaten with sour foods.

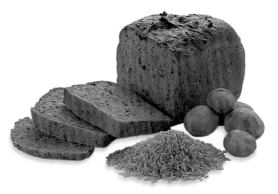

Heavy foods

Bread, grains, and other heavy foods should form about three-quarters of your diet.

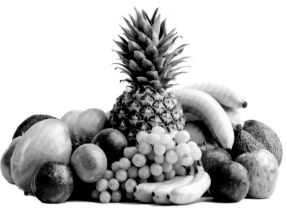

To be eaten alone
*Different types of fruit can be
mixed, but fruit should always
be eaten on its own.*

Mealtime habits
Because the digestive system is
so central to Ayurvedic philosophy,
it is important to consider carefully
what you are eating and what you
are doing while you eat. Watching
television or reading a book while
eating is strongly discouraged.

Pure nourishment
Different food types are
recommended for different
doshas, but the most vital thing is
to eat fresh, unprocessed foods
as often as possible, to prevent
the build-up of toxins in the body.

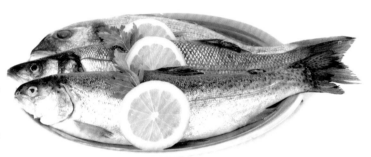

Fish
*Fish is a healthy part of an
Ayurvedic diet, but should not
be cooked with milk.*

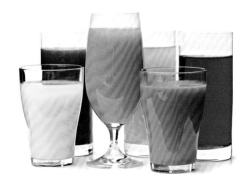

Refreshments
*Drink plenty of liquids, but do
not have anything other than
small sips of water with meals.*

General Guidelines
for an Ayurvedic Diet

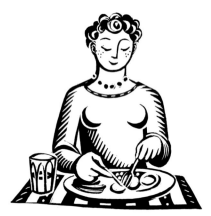

Eat with care

*Your choice of food and eating
habits will help to ensure healthy
digestion and balanced doshas.*

Overall, a good diet will allow
for the occasional indiscretion.
Ayurvedic practitioners
recommend a general revision of your
eating habits around the guidelines listed
on this page, to ensure that your digestive
system works efficiently. Remember that
this isn't intended as a short-term diet, but
as a new way of eating that will affect
your health and vitality in the future.

Time to eat

It is best to allow three to six hours
between mealtimes, to give your
system time to digest the previous meal
properly—snacking should not usually
be necessary if you are eating well. The
largest meal of the day should be lunch,
and it should take place between 12 and
1pm. Dinner should be a lighter meal
and is best eaten no later than 7.30 pm.

Always eat at a moderate pace—not
too quickly, and not too slowly. Do not
eat when you are nervous, angry, or
frightened, as any emotional state is not
conducive to good digestion. Similarly,
do not drink when you are hungry or
eat when you are thirsty. Avoid drinking
anything more than small sips of water
with your meals.

Choosing food

When you buy food, consider the seasons
(see pages 136–37) and the doshas,
and choose produce of good quality—
fresh foods are best when they have been

produced locally. Meals should contain at least three of the six basic tastes (see pages 158–61), and be freshly prepared and warmed whenever possible. Use spices in your cooking to promote good digestion.

Fruits are best eaten on their own, and make an ideal food for breakfast. Different types of fruit can be mixed, but fruit should not be mixed with other types of food.

Sour dairy foods such as yogurt should not be eaten at the same time (or in the same meal) as sweet dairy produce, such as milk and cream. Do not eat dairy produce with starches.

Raw foods, such as salads, should not be eaten at the same time as you eat cooked foods.

Good Hygiene

Make the environments in which you prepare and eat your food pleasant, and always keep both your kitchen and dining room clean.

TASTES & THE DOSHAS

The energies of the six tastes act directly on the doshas, and can be used to readjust an unbalanced body into a balanced state. A dosha can be increased or decreased according to the specific properties of the taste. This will affect body processes—for example, speeding them up or slowing them down, or heating or cooling them. A balanced diet should be composed of the six tastes, but predominantly the three tastes that suit your constitution.

Which food?

Choose foods that reduce the energy of your predominant dosha and fortify your secondary or subsidiary dosha. For example, if you are a kapha type, you should eat mainly foods that reduce kapha and strengthen vata and pitta.

The general rules are:
- Sweet, sour, and salty tastes will increase kapha and decrease vata.
- Pungent, bitter, and astringent tastes increase vata and decrease kapha.
- Sour, salty, and pungent tastes increase pitta.
- Sweet, bitter, and astringent tastes decrease pitta.

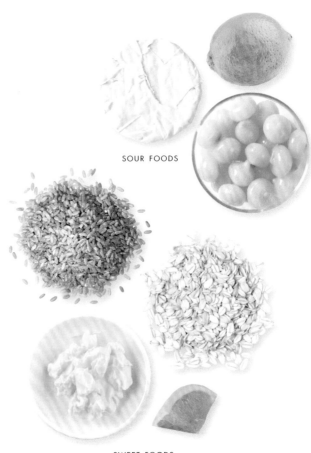

SOUR FOODS

Sweet & sour foods

Sweet foods will alleviate vata and pitta, and increase kapha energy, while sour foods increase pitta and kapha.

SWEET FOODS

Moisture & dryness
Tastes have qualities that add or decrease moisture in the body: pungent, bitter, and astringent tastes are drying, while sweet, salty, and sour are moistening. One of the qualities of vata is dryness, so when in excess vata, choose tastes that are moistening.

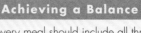

Achieving a Balance
Ideally every meal should include all three rasas that alleviate your dosha, as this will ensure a balancing effect on the three vital energies (doshas) of vata, pitta, and kapha.

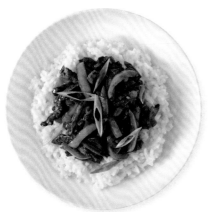

Vata
Sweet and sour stir-fried beef with vegetables combines two of the best tastes for vata types.

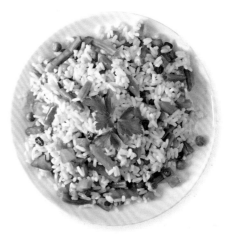

Pitta
Rice, fish, and salad suit pitta types, who benefit from sweet, bitter, and astringent tastes.

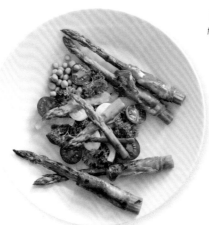

Kapha
Astringent asparagus is good for kaphas, who should also eat pungent and bitter foods.

159

The Six Tastes

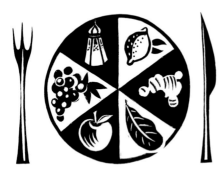

Which taste?

Each of the doshas is affected by the six tastes, which can either aggravate or alleviate health problems.

The Sanskrit word for taste is *rasa*, meaning "essential part" or "essence." This gives us some idea of the importance of taste in Ayurvedic medicine. Rasa reflects the true qualities of a plant or food, and the taste of anything is always taken into consideration.

Taste stimulates the nervous system and also affects all of the systems of the body. It enlivens prana (our living energy) and awakens the mind. Furthermore, through taste, the agni (metabolic fire) is stimulated and proper digestion is encouraged.

Taste	Elements	Foods
SWEET	Earth and water	Barley, butter, cabbage, cream, fruits such as pears and bananas, ghee, grapes, lentils, milk, oats, oils such as sesame, onions, peas, rice, rye, starches, sugar, wheat
SALTY	Fire and water	Table or sea salt
SOUR	Earth and fire	Cheeses, fruits such as citrus fruits, morello cherries, and rosehips, pickles, vinegars, yogurt
PUNGENT	Fire and air	Black pepper, caraway, chamomile, chile, cinnamon, cumin, dill, ginger, mustard, nutmeg, parsley, radishes, bell peppers
BITTER	Ether and air	Brussels sprouts, coffee, herbs such as fenugreek and goldenseal, horse chestnut, nettles, rhubarb, spinach and other leafy greens, turmeric
ASTRINGENT	Earth and air	Apples, asparagus, eggplants, bananas, beans, broccoli, cauliflower, celery, endive, fennel, herbs such as witch hazel, pears

Tastes & their properties

Food is categorized into six tastes in Ayurveda—sweet, salty, sour, pungent, bitter, and astringent. Each is composed of two basic elements and has its own series of characteristics and properties. Foods with sweet tastes, such as sugar and cream, add strength and have a laxative and tonic effect on the body. Salt and other foods with salty tastes are stimulating, soothe the membranes, and also have a laxative effect.

Sour tastes, found in citrus fruits and pickles, are stimulating, and pungent tastes, which many spices have, are diuretic, stimulating, diaphoretic, and decongestant. Bitter tastes are diuretic, detoxifying, and balancing—spinach and other leafy greens are all bitter. Astringent tastes have a contracting effect on mind and body and mop up excess secretions. Foods that have astringent tastes include cauliflower and broccoli.

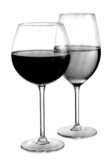

Drinking wine
Alcohol is not considered a part of a healthy Ayurvedic diet, and it should be drunk on rare occasions or not at all.

FOOD & THE SEASONS Appetite and digestive function will vary according to the season. Furthermore, seasons are dominated by one of the three doshas (see pages 136–37), which will also affect what should be eaten. No foods are definitely off the list in specific seasons, but the foods suggested here are those that will work toward balancing your diet in that season. For example, sweet, astringent, and bitter tastes will help to balance pitta in summer.

Kapha (spring)
Most people will require less food in the spring than they do in the winter. Some Ayurvedic practitioners believe that healthy people should fast for one day every week during this period (see pages 180–81).
- Concentrate on pungent, bitter, and astringent tastes.
- Avoid foods that have a high acid content.
- Sweet foods should be avoided because the body finds it difficult to cope with extra calories during this time.
- Sleep only at night and avoid taking daytime naps.

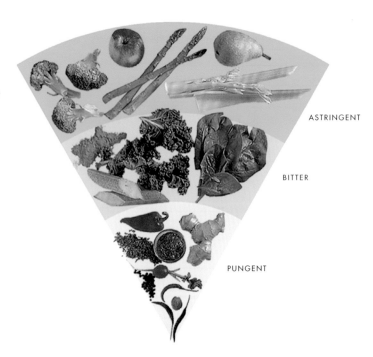

ASTRINGENT

BITTER

PUNGENT

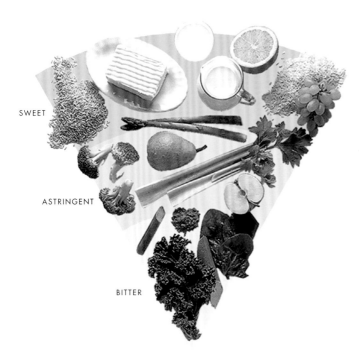

SWEET

ASTRINGENT

BITTER

Pitta (summer)

In summer, foods should be mostly warm to cool rather than very hot.

- Cold, soft foods will cool the body. Avoid any heat-producing foods.
- Favor the sweet, bitter, and astringent tastes.
- Cook only sparingly with cheese, yogurt, tomatoes, lemon, or pungent spices.
- Start and end meals with sweet-tasting food.
- Alcohol should be avoided or diluted.

Vata (fall/winter)

During the winter, your digestive function increases and heavier foods can be digested more easily as your metabolism will be increased. Most people find they can consume the increased quantities of food required by the body (and vata) during the colder months.

- Favor the sweet, sour, and salty tastes.
- Choose comforting foods, such as milk, meat, honey, oil, and rice, which are appropriate for the season.
- Well-cooked, oily foods are also appropriate.

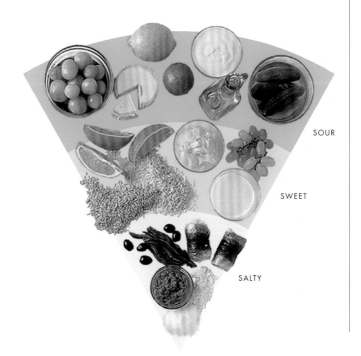

SOUR

SWEET

SALTY

Food Categories

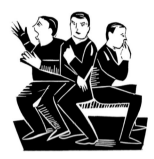

Food for health

For maximum vitality, all the doshas should include as high a proportion of sattvic foods as possible in their diets.

In Ayurveda, food is broken into three main categories—the same ones that define the mind (see page 52–53). These are sattvic, rajasic, and tamasic, or pure, stimulating, and ignorant. The categories also represent high, medium, and low quality.

At most times of your life, you should aim to eat largely sattvic foods, which are health-giving. This is particularly important when you are entering the older vata years (see pages 138–39). A sattvic diet will promote longevity and vitality when it is used correctly.

Sattvic food

These foods should be the highest quality available and include fresh fruit and vegetables, dried fruit, salads, lentils, plain yogurt, milk, fresh butter, wheat, rye, barley, hazelnuts, almonds, wholegrain rice, and honey. These types of food help to maintain your physical health and to improve your sense of well-being. Through this, your emotional health and spirit will be positively affected. Sattvic foods are recommended to keep us young.

Rajasic food

This type of food is considered to be of medium quality, even if the ingredients are pure and unadulterated. These foods are rich in protein and encourage energy. Rajasic foods include sugar, meat, cheese, fish, fried foods, eggs, potatoes, and other root vegetables. Candies are also rajasic.

Because some of these foods may have been processed, they are less kind to the mind and the body. Up until the age of about 45, these foods are acceptable in smaller quantities than the sattvic foods, but after that, when the vata years approach, you will need to release all extra energy for reducing accumulated toxins and ama.

Tamasic food

There is little doubt that all of us consume these foods, which include dried (except dried fruit), canned, contaminated, processed, and junk food. Alcohol is tamasic, as are potato chips, burgers, prepared meals, and anything else that has preservatives and flavor enhancers. Anything that is completely processed will be tamasic.

What do these foods do? Generally, they damage health on all levels by causing a physical imbalance that impairs emotional and mental functioning. Through this imbalance, they also damage spiritual health.

State of Mind

The foods you eat will affect your mood. Therefore, choosing sattvic foods over tamasic foods will affect your sense of well-being.

A vata diet
If you are vata, aim for a diet that has plenty of foods that are low in vata.

FOOD & THE DOSHAS All foods have vata, pitta, and kapha
qualities, and your diet should be based around your constitutional type. The foods
suggested over the next few pages can be used to balance your constitutional type
or to reduce a dosha if it is causing imbalance. It can be difficult to assess what foods
are right, particularly if you have a specific health condition which presents different
requirements. It's a good idea to see an Ayurvedic practitioner for assistance.

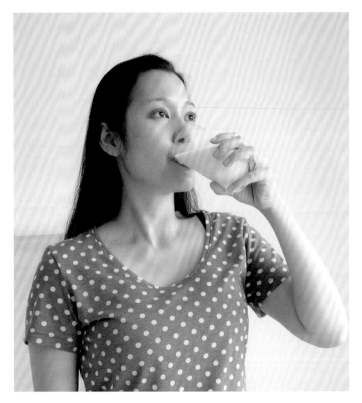

Vata types
People who are vata—or those attempting to reduce vata—should avoid all fried foods and make sure that they eat at regular intervals. Dryness is a characteristic of vata. To achieve balance, vata types should eat heavy, oily, hot foods and stick to salty, sour, and sweet tastes.

Balancing drinks
What you drink is important too. Choose drinks that help to balance your doshas.

Recommended Foods for Vata Types

• Herbs & spices
Basil, bay, black mustard, cardamom, cloves, coriander, cumin, dill, fennel, fresh ginger, marjoram, mint, nutmeg, oregano, paprika, parsley, peppermint, spearmint, tarragon, thyme, turmeric, vanilla

• Grains & seeds
Oats (cooked), pumpkin seeds, quinoa, rice, sesame seeds, sprouted wheat bread, sunflower seeds, wheat

• Beans & legumes
Lentils, mung dhal, beancurd

• Nuts
Almonds, brazil nuts, cashews, coconut, hazelnuts, macadamias, pecans, pine nuts, pistachios, walnuts

• Meat & fish
Beef, chicken, duck, shellfish, shrimp, turkey. Vatas may benefit from eating plenty of meat and fish

• Vegetables
Artichokes, asparagus, beet, carrots, cucumbers, green beans, leeks, okra, onions, parsnips, pumpkins, radishes, rutabaga, spinach (cooked), sweet potatoes, tomatoes (cooked), watercress, zucchini

• Fruit
Apricots, avocados, bananas, berries, cherries, dates, fresh figs, grapefruit, grapes, lemons, limes, mangoes, melons, oranges, peaches, pineapples, plums, rhubarb, strawberries

• Dairy produce
Cottage cheese, eggs, cow's milk, eggs, goat cheese, goat milk

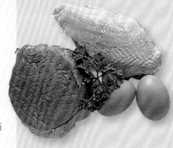

• Oils
Sesame

• Drinks
Fruit juices, spice teas, vegetables juice, warm milk, warm water

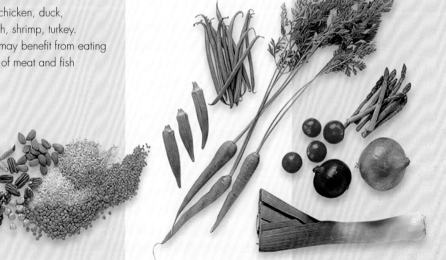

Pitta

A pitta diet

Pitta types need cooling down, and their fire is often exacerbated in hot weather.

Pitta types should avoid all hot, spicy, and sour foods, as they will aggravate this dosha. You should also try to avoid fried foods. Eat more raw than cooked foods whenever possible, and stick to vegetarian food as often as you can. The pitta dosha is hot, which is why pitta types should eat mainly cool, refreshing foods, particularly in summer.

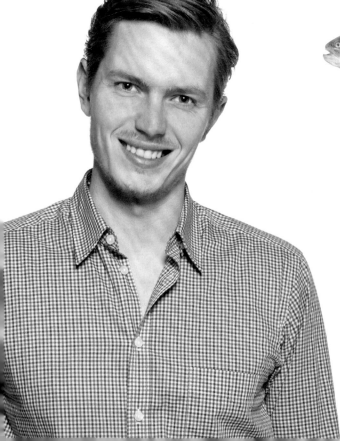

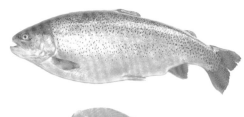

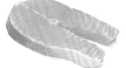

Freshwater fish

Choose freshwater rather than sea fish, and avoid deep-frying, batters, and breadcrumbs.

Food for health

Pitta people should eat plenty of salads, fruits, and vegetables. But choose carefully: some fruits and vegetables increase pitta.

Recommended Foods for Pitta Types

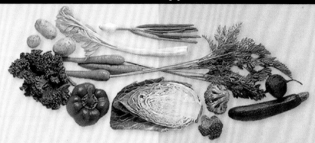

- **Herbs & spices**
Aloe vera juice, basil, cinnamon, coriander, cumin, dill, dulse, fennel, fresh ginger, mint leaves, spearmint.

- **Grains & seeds**
Barley, basmati rice, flax seeds, psyllium seeds, rice cakes, sunflower seeds, wheat, wheat bran, white rice

- **Beans & legumes**
Adzuki beans, beancurd, black beans, black-eye peas, garbanzo beans, kidney beans, lentils, lima beans, mung beans, pinto beans, soy beans, split peas

- **Nuts**
Almonds, coconuts

- **Meat & fish**
Chicken, freshwater fish, rabbit, turkey, venison

- **Vegetables**
Artichokes, asparagus, broccoli, Brussels sprouts, butternut squash, cabbage, carrots, cauliflower, cucumber, celery, fennel, green beans, green bell peppers, Jerusalem artichokes, kale, leafy greens, leeks, lettuce, mushrooms, onions (cooked), parsnips, peas, potatoes, pumpkins, rutabaga, spinach (cooked), sweet potatoes, winter squash, zucchini

- **Fruit**
Apples, apricots, avocados, berries, cherries, dates, figs, grapefruit, mangoes, melons, oranges, pears, pineapples, plums, pomegranates, prunes, quince, raisins, red grapes, watermelon

- **Dairy produce**
Cottage and soft cheese, cows' milk, diluted yogurt, ghee, goat milk, sweet butter

- **Oils**
Olive, sunflower, soy, walnut

- **Drinks**
Cool water, milk, milkshakes, fruit juices, vegetable bouillon, teas made of alfalfa, comfrey, dandelion, hibiscus, mint

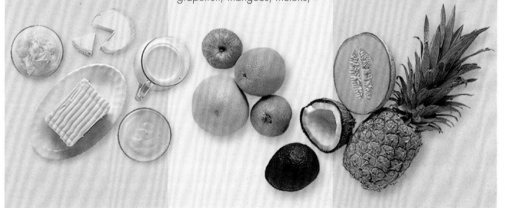

A kapha diet

Kapha types respond best to heating and cooked foods, and should eat cooling foods only in moderation, except in summer.

KAPHA
Kapha people should eat mostly cooked food, with the occasional salad. Avoid fats and oils unless they are hot and spicy. Dairy produce, and sweet, sour, and salty tastes will aggravate kapha. Many kaphas do not respond well to wheat or animal products. Pungent, bitter, astringent tastes have a balancing effect on kapha.

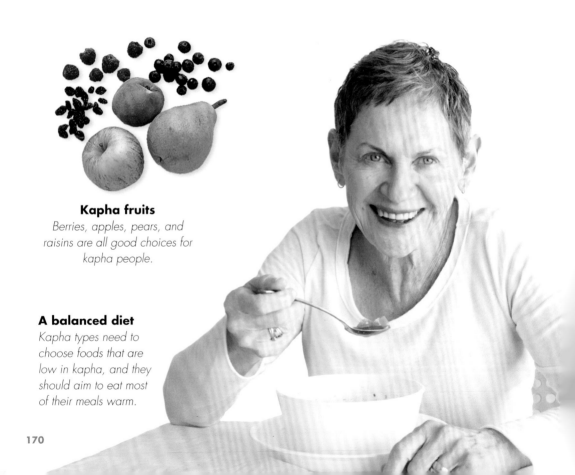

Kapha fruits
Berries, apples, pears, and raisins are all good choices for kapha people.

A balanced diet
Kapha types need to choose foods that are low in kapha, and they should aim to eat most of their meals warm.

Recommended Foods for Kapha Types

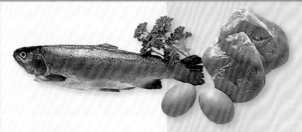

• **Herbs & spices**
Black pepper or pippali, chile pepper, coriander, dry ginger, garlic, horseradish, mint leaves, mustard, onions, parsley, radishes; any other hot spices

• **Grains & seeds**
Barley, buckwheat, corn, couscous, oatbran, polenta, plain popcorn, rye, sprouted wheat bread, toasted pumpkin and sunflower seeds

• **Beans & legumes**
Adzuki beans, black-eye peas, garbanzo beans, lima beans, pinto beans, red lentils, split peas, tempeh

• **Meat & fish**
Eggs, freshwater fish, turkey, rabbit, shrimp, venison

• **Vegetables**
Artichokes, asparagus, beet, bell peppers, broccoli, Brussels sprouts, cabbage, carrots, cauliflower, corn, eggplant, fennel, green beans, kale, leeks, lettuce, mushrooms, okra, onions, peas, potatoes radishes, rutabaga, spinach, turnips, watercress

• **Fruit**
Apples, apricots, berries, cherries, cranberries, peaches, pears, pomegranates, prunes, raisins

• **Dairy produce**
Low-fat cows' milk, goat milk, (or soy milk)

• **Oils**
Mustard, safflower, sunflower

• **Drinks**
Carrot juice and other vegetable juices, cranberry juice, grape juice, mango juice, spice teas: endive, cinnamon, dandelion

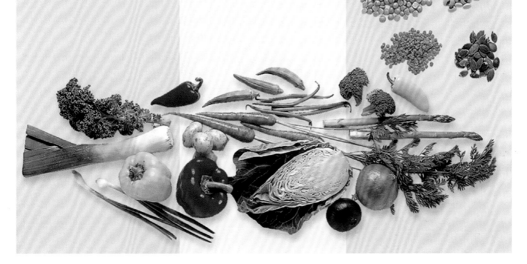

Agni—Metabolic Fire

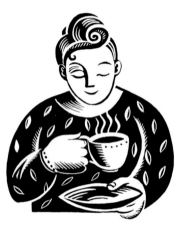

The fire within
Agni equates to metabolism in Western terms. In Ayurveda, good digestion and metabolism are essential for health.

Agni is the digestive fire which, when working normally, maintains normality in all functions. As well as describing the digestive functions, it also covers the other body parts or forces that are involved in the process of consuming, converting, and eliminating food, including the pancreas, gallbladder, liver, and salivary glands. Unbalanced agni is caused by imbalances in the doshas, and such actions as eating and drinking too much of the wrong types of foods and repressing emotions rather than releasing them.

Agni that is affected by too much kapha can slow the digestive process, making you feel heavy and sluggish, while too much vata can lead to gas, cramps, and alternating constipation and diarrhea. Agni also ensures that the three malas (see pages 64–65) are working effectively.

In Ayurveda, good digestion is the key to good health. Poor digestion produces ama—a toxicity believed to cause illness. Ama is seen in the body as a white coating on the tongue, but it can also line the colon and clog blood vessels. Ama occurs when the metabolism is impaired due to an imbalance of agni.

Many factors can influence the quality of agni in your body. Eating too much or too often, or consuming heavy meals, unhealthy food, or too much protein in the evening can diminish the fire and cause it to lose its intensity. Eating a main meal in the evening can also weaken agni, as can reading, watching television, or arguing while you are eating.

Stimulating agni

Certain foods and spices can be used to stimulate the digestion.

• Ginger helps to stabilize agni in every constitutional type. Fresh ginger is the best source. Try drinking a cup of ginger tea before meals.

• Ghee, or clarified butter, strengthens agni without inflaming pitta (the fiery dosha). You can use it as an alternative to ordinary butter.

• Various spices improve agni. These include black pepper, cloves, cardamom, mustard, horseradish, cayenne pepper, and cinnamon.

A Healthy Force

When agni is working at its optimum level, body cells are able to absorb nourishment, waste products are burned off, and we digest our food efficiently. Overall good health and weight are among the beneficial results.

APPETITE

When your mind, body, and spirit are in balance, you will achieve a natural, healthy appetite. As your body becomes accustomed to the routine of eating foods that work to balance the vital energies, you will find that you are hungry only at mealtimes. When you get hungry between good, healthy meals, you may consider this hunger to be a symptom of imbalance.

Fuel for the body

When you provide your body with healthy meals, you should find that snacking is no longer necessary.

Doshas & Appetite

Each of the constitutional types has an appetite for different types of food, and that appetite may be big or small, or somewhere in between.

- Kapha types have a slow, steady appetite and a regular, steady digestion. They take in small quantities of food because of their efficient digestions.

- Vata types have variable appetite and digestion. They are attracted to astringent foods such as raw vegetables, but their constitution is balanced by warm, cooked foods and sweet, sour, and salty tastes.

- Those with pitta-dominant constitutions have strong metabolisms, good digestions, and strong appetites. They like plenty of food and liquids, and love hot spices and cold drinks. Pitta is balanced by sweet, bitter, and astringent tastes.

Fresh is best

An Ayurvedic diet is basically healthy, with plenty of fresh, whole foods. Even in Western terms, this will improve the digestion. Imbalanced agni is often caused by eating and drinking too much of the wrong thing.

Causes of Imbalance

When you do not eat regularly, or when you eat poor-quality food, you can upset the balance of the doshas.

- An erratic appetite, which is called *vishamagni*, puts the vata dosha out of equilibrium and causes very slow digestion as well as the following symptoms: abdominal bloating and heaviness, abdominal discomfort, constipation, diarrhea, flatulence, and gurgling sounds.

- Overeating, called *thikshanangi*, can cause the pitta dosha to become unbalanced, creating feelings of intense hunger. This in turn can cause you to eat too much in a short period of time, or cause rapid digestion, sweating while eating, or an impaired sense of taste and smell.

- Lack of appetite, which is called *mandagni*, unbalances kapha energy, and can prevent the digestion from working properly. It can also cause abdominal pains, slow down the agni, affect respiration, cause nausea and even vomiting, and lead to general feelings of ill health and fatigue.

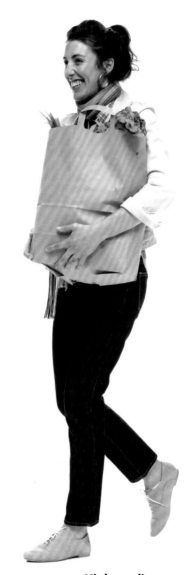

High quality
Choosing sattvic foods will help to balance the doshas and thus regulate the appetite.

The Causes of Excess Weight

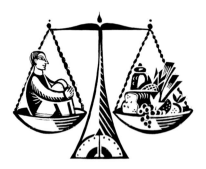

Finding a balance
You are more likely to reach and maintain your natural weight if you eat a balanced Ayurvedic diet.

When you adopt an Ayurvedic lifestyle and eat foods according to your dosha and your current level of health and well-being, your weight will stabilize at its natural level.

Excess weight is a sign of imbalance within the body, and there is a variety of tools that you can use in order to find the weight that is right for you. Ayurveda classifies certain health problems, including obesity, as "diseases of affluence." The affluent state of mind is defined as one in which someone believes that he or she has time and money to waste. Remember also that your ideal weight will be one which is appropriate for your constitution. Kapha women should not, therefore, expect to be extremely thin, while vata types may be thinner than average. In Ayurveda, it is generally considered better to be too thin than too fat; however, too little fat can weaken immunity.

Dosha imbalances

There are various reasons for being overweight, according to Ayurveda.

When there is extreme overeating, both vata and pitta doshas are unbalanced. Low levels of vata mean that the thyroid doesn't function properly and the metabolism becomes sluggish. When pitta is reduced, kapha accumulates in the fatty cells. Water retention, a cause of obesity in some cases, is believed to result from a dosha imbalance that allows kapha to become overdominant.

If there is inadequate vata energy to move the lymph around the body, toxins can build up, causing excess weight.

If you are following the wrong kind of diet (for example, a tamasic diet, see pages 164–65), you may be eating foods that cause food addictions or cravings. Junk food has a tendency to do this. If you are overweight and cannot see a reason why you are unable to shift the pounds, take a look at the types of food that you are eating.

Aids to Weight Control

• *Guggul* is highly recommended in all of the ancient texts of Ayurveda to control obesity, however it should not be consumed during pregnancy.

• *Triphala choornam, triphala guggul,* and *medohar guggul* are multi-herb preparations that are used to control excess weight.

• *Karela* (bitter melon) is a wonderful vegetable for controlling weight. It should be cooked according to Ayurvedic principles.

YOUR IDEAL WEIGHT

Ayurveda aims to balance your weight, and that means ensuring that your weight is healthy for your constitutional type. Being underweight is taken as seriously as being overweight in Ayurveda since it also reflects an imbalance of the doshas. When you see an Ayurvedic practitioner, you will not be prescribed drugs to encourage you to lose or gain pounds, although there are some herbal remedies that help (see page 177). Instead, you will be offered advice on how to adopt a healthy lifestyle by following a balanced and healthy diet.

Balancing the doshas

The first step in reaching your natural weight is to balance your doshas by a gradual change to your diet. Excess kapha can result in obesity, so if you have a tendency to be overweight, consider eating foods that reduce kapha (see page 171). See a practitioner for advice since this isn't as straightforward as it seems—for example, going on an anti-kapha diet when you are vata-provoked could throw you further off balance.

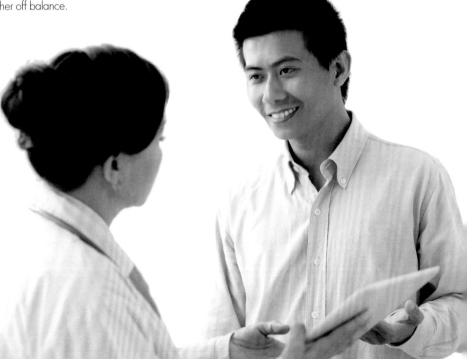

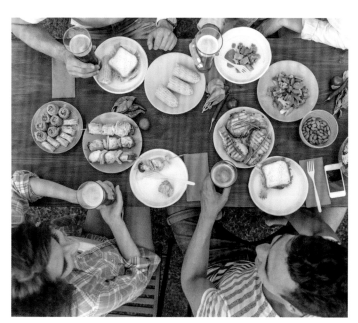

Your state of mind

Many Ayurvedic practitioners suggest that in order to lose pounds and stay at a healthy weight, you need to adopt a healthily austere state of mind. What this means is recognizing that waste of any kind is just that—wasteful. If you are overweight, your goal should be to transform yourself, not just to lose weight but to improve your mental and emotional state. This will be a slower process, but in weight loss, as in other aspects of Ayurvedic medicine, hasty action normally doesn't go very far.

When to eat

Before eating, consider these guidelines. Eat only when you need to satisfy hunger. If you are not hungry, don't eat. Sit down while you are eating and do nothing else while you are having your meal—no reading, telephone calls, or talking, for example.

Eggs
increase
kapha

Water retention

An overabundance of kapha foods, such as eggs, in your diet can lead to water retention.

Fasting

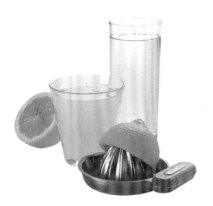

Drinks for fasting
Choose vegetable juices or herbal teas appropriate for your dosha. Water and lemon juice aid detoxification.

F asting is an important part of Ayurvedic practice and can bring great benefits. It is an effective treatment for clearing and balancing the system, and also for treating many diseases because it rids the body of toxins and stirs up the agni, or metabolic fire.

Some Ayurvedic practitioners recommend that normal, healthy people fast for one day a week. However, a springtime fast is often enough to keep toxins at bay. Detoxification is a major part of Ayurvedic medicine, and there are other means of ridding the body of toxins other than fasting, such as massage (see page 78). When you are fasting, your agni will become very strong, and without food to divert its energies, it will burn away toxins present in the body.

A variety of different fasts can be undertaken. Water fasts or fasts using teas, juices, and broths are all acceptable. It is extremely important, however, to ensure that you are healthy enough to fast before you begin. This means seeing an Ayurvedic practitioner, or your own doctor to check before you start.

Plenty of liquids

Ensure that you drink between one and two liters of liquid every day that you are fasting. The following drinks are acceptable on fasting days: water (fresh, filtered, or spring water), herbal teas, such as raspberry or ginseng, vegetable juices, and lemon juice and water.

Fruit juices are not recommended because they encourage ama when they are taken during fasts, although lemon juice is acceptable. Furthermore, fruit juices may play havoc with your blood-sugar levels.

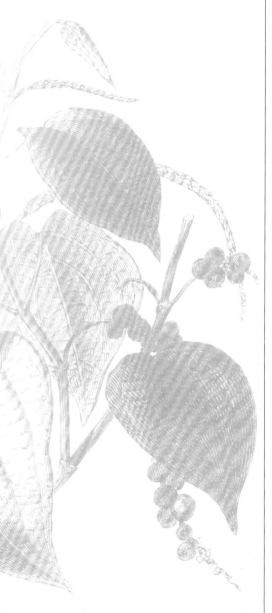

Alternative herbal teas

Herbs that can be taken in the form of a tea during fasts also include long pepper, black pepper, cayenne, ginger, basil, and cardamom. These will help with the elimination process.

Do not add these teas or herbs to your diet, however, unless you have consulted an Ayurvedic practitioner beforehand. You can also purchase prepackaged Ayurvedic teas to aid with detoxification from health-food stores.

How Long Should I Fast?

Kapha types may benefit from a longer period of fasting—up to a week, for example. Vata and pitta people should never fast for longer than three days at a time. Again, it is essential not to start fasting before checking your state of health with a registered Ayurvedic or Western physician.

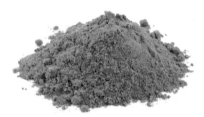

Good for all
Turmeric is one spice that can help all three doshas. Add it to your food two or three times a week, or more often if you like.

FOOD AS MEDICINE
Even the healthiest lifestyle and diet may be unable to prevent imbalance from setting in at times. Furthermore, you may find that although you are changing your habits and your energies are beginning to find their equilibrium, there may be periods when you may feel worse. On the path to good health, you can use a variety of different spices and foods to help in the balancing process, and restore a feeling of well-being to the body, mind, and spirit.

Ginger
Dried ginger balances all three doshas when it is taken in moderation. Fresh ginger can increase pitta. Ginger encourages appetite, intensifies agni, relieves bloating and abdominal distension, prevents motion sickness, and helps chronic diarrhea.

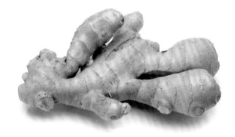

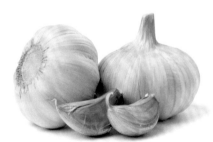

Garlic
Vata or kapha imbalances are relieved by garlic, which improves digestion, circulation, and tissue nutrition, kills harmful bacteria, promotes memory, and helps dry-skin conditions, colic, coughs, heart problems, asthma, and indigestion.

Turmeric

Used externally and internally, turmeric purifies the blood and the mind, and balances the three doshas. It also keeps the blood cool. When applied to wounds, it slows any bleeding. As a natural antibiotic, it protects the intestinal flora and promotes the production of bile.

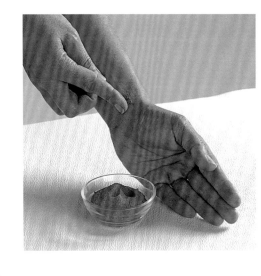

Onions

Heart-stimulating onions promote the production of bile and reduce blood-sugar levels. The fresh juice of one medium-sized red onion makes a good heart tonic when taken in the morning with a tablespoon of honey. Smelling a crushed onion (left) can ease headaches and nausea.

A Diet for Your Constitution

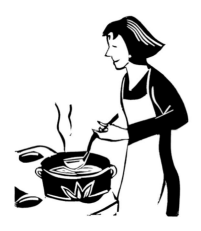

Everyone is unique
Your diet should be altered to reflect your personal requirements and dosha.

There may seem to be a great deal of complicated theory behind an Ayurvedic diet, and you may feel that you need the help of a qualified practitioner before you embark on a new eating program. However, there are a number of basic principles that can help to make the process easier to understand and implement.

First of all, choose foods that will balance or pacify your predominant doshas and stimulate the other doshas. If you are a kapha type, this means choosing foods that reduce kapha in the body and stimulate pitta and vata. Pitta types should choose food that pacify pitta and stimulate kapha and vata, while vata types should choose foods that pacify vata and stimulate kapha and pitta. Foods for each dosha are listed on pages 166–71.

Adjust your diet to suit the time of year. The seasons are important to your overall diet, and you will need to choose foods that are appropriate for your constitutional type, depending on the time of year.

Vata

Choose nourishing, heavy, oily, and hot foods. Rice, pasta, warm milk, cream, and warm bread will all help to balance the dosha. Cold foods, such as salads, raw vegetables, or cold drinks, intensify vata so should be avoided. Choose salty, sour, and sweet tastes. Eat warm, cooked, easily digestible meals to regulate agni.

Pitta

Choose cool, refreshing foods, particularly in the summer. Avoid anything that increases heat, including salt, oil, and pungent seasonings and foods. Include some bitter and astringent tastes in your diet, to curb the appetite. Do not skip meals.

Kapha

Avoid foods that are heavy, fatty, or cold. If you eat too much, you will become energetically unbalanced. Eat low-fat, lightly cooked dishes with plenty of fresh fruit and raw vegetables. The key words for kapha are light, dry, and hot. Pungent, bitter and astringent tastes balance kapha. Kapha is the one dosha that can afford to miss meals.

See a Practitioner

Diet is important in Ayurveda, and you may need the guidance of a practitioner to ensure that you are getting what you need, according to your health, your dosha, and other factors.

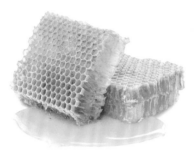

Healing honey
Eating plenty of honey during the winter months helps to prevent toxic build-up.

DETOXIFYING
Food and drink are crucially important in Ayurveda, and many foods have the additional ability to help the body in its detoxification process. Detoxification is a process that should be undertaken regularly, in order to keep the doshas in balance. Detoxification eliminates the influence of negative doshas and rids the body of accumulated ama.

Massage
As part of your detoxification program, consider incorporating self-massage into your morning routine, using oils that are appropriate for your dosha type. Massage moves the toxins from beneath the skin and helps the body to eliminate them. When you follow your massage with a hot bath, you will be able to sweat out the impurities. Massage also unblocks lymphatic circulation.

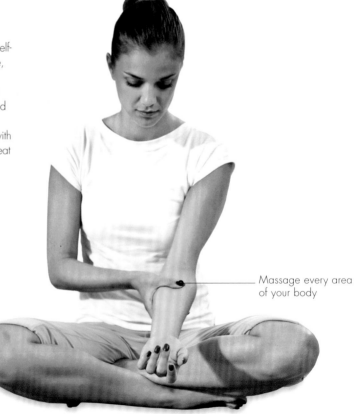

Massage every area of your body

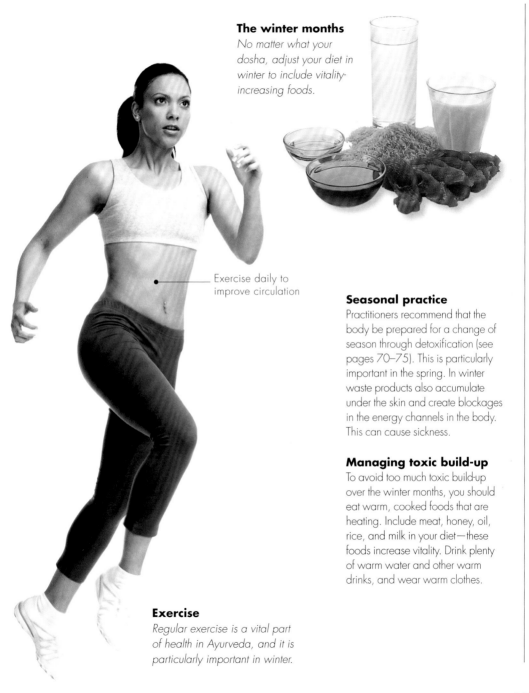

The winter months

No matter what your dosha, adjust your diet in winter to include vitality-increasing foods.

Exercise daily to improve circulation

Seasonal practice

Practitioners recommend that the body be prepared for a change of season through detoxification (see pages 70–75). This is particularly important in the spring. In winter waste products also accumulate under the skin and create blockages in the energy channels in the body. This can cause sickness.

Managing toxic build-up

To avoid too much toxic build-up over the winter months, you should eat warm, cooked foods that are heating. Include meat, honey, oil, rice, and milk in your diet—these foods increase vitality. Drink plenty of warm water and other warm drinks, and wear warm clothes.

Exercise

Regular exercise is a vital part of health in Ayurveda, and it is particularly important in winter.

187

Detoxification at Home

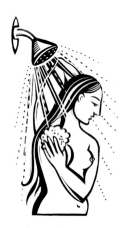

Ama therapy
Regular self-detoxification can improve health and well-being and help to ward off disease.

Self-detoxification is called ama therapy, as it aims to detoxify the body of ama, which is metabolic waste, environmental pollution, and undigested food. A build-up of ama in the body can block channels and cause serious illness, and general feelings of ill health and fatigue. Ama can also be caused by unresolved emotional issues, and you will find that any detoxification program will work better if you deal with these and include a little meditation as part of your therapy.

Removing obstructions

The courses of action recommended in this book will work more effectively if you detoxify first. When you eliminate toxins and waste products, your energy will travel more easily throughout the body, working to heal, balance, and restore. Without detoxification, even the best therapies can be trapped by obstructions caused by ama. While you are detoxifying, ensure that you take regular warm baths to remove the toxins and bacteria from the pores, and to allow the internal toxins to be eliminated more effectively.

Diet detox

The following ama-reducing diet can be practiced for five to ten days. However, you should always check with your doctor before adopting any major changes to your diet.

Morning Drink a glass of warm water with two tablespoons of fresh lemon juice and two tablespoons of honey. Avoid eating if you can, but if you are hungry, try a glass of fresh fruit juice.

Lunch Have a light, warm meal. Try to eat fresh, whole foods that are appropriate to your dosha type. Eat only as much as you need. Tamasic foods (see page 165) should be avoided during this detoxification program. Stick with sattvic foods. This is your biggest meal of the day. Sit quietly while you eat.

Dinner Avoid eating in the evening if you can. If you are hungry, have a little soup with rice and vegetables, or simply some fruit juice. Again, ensure that anything you eat is sattvic in nature.

If you are hungry between meals, drink fresh vegetable juice. Carrot juice is particularly good. Drink warm water throughout the day to cleanse. When you have finished the diet, introduce other foods. Do not go back to your old eating habits, and continue to eat as many sattvic foods as you can.

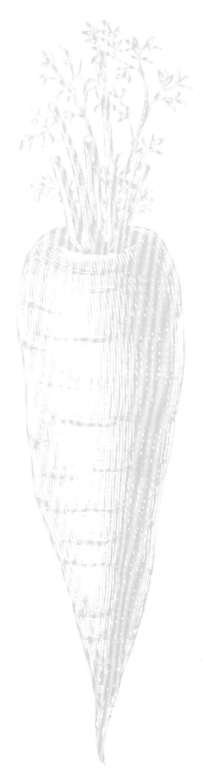

Vegetables

Freshly squeezed and lightly cooked fresh vegetables are important in detoxification, and should form part of your daily diet.

PRACTITIONER-LED OR SELF-HELP?

As you have seen, Ayurveda is more than just a medical system. It involves making changes to almost every aspect of your lifestyle and working toward health that is bountiful, vital, and permanent. No matter how well you take care of yourself, however, there are times when medical treatment may be necessary. This is when an Ayurvedic practitioner will be invaluable. Apart from suggesting lifestyle changes, he or she will offer a variety of treatments (some of which have been described in this book) in order to balance your health, prevent illness, and treat health conditions when they arise. However, there is also plenty you can do to treat yourself at home, before and after seeing a physician. This section tells you what to expect when you see a practitioner and summarizes what you can do to treat yourself.

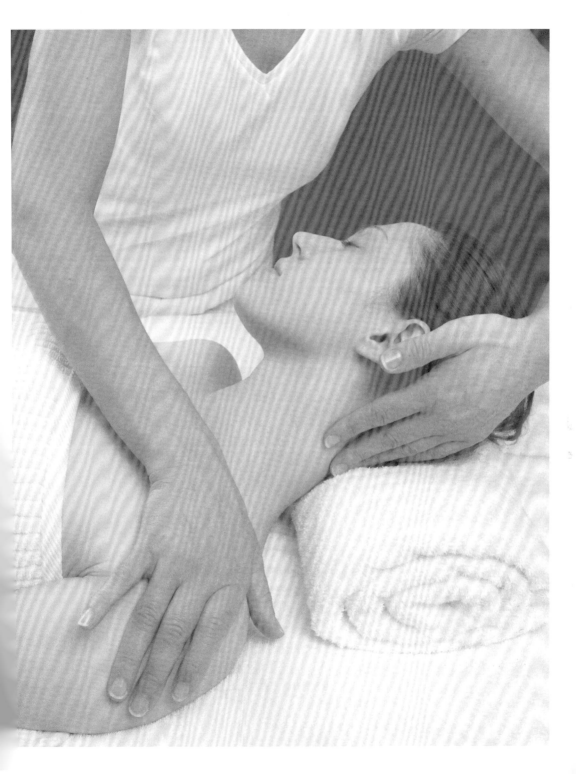

Seeing a Practitioner

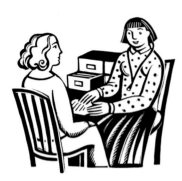

Consultation
*When you see a practitioner,
be prepared to be open about
your symptoms and habits.*

Ayurvedic practitioners treat every patient differently, and as a result, they need to know a great deal about you and your lifestyle before treatment can begin. The first thing a practitioner will do is assess your constitutional type (see pages 196–97). In general, most practitioners do this simply by looking at you and checking various signs.

Because it is a complete system of medicine, practitioners say that Ayurvedic medicine can help with any problem, whether it is mental, physical, or emotional. Ayurveda is particularly beneficial for digestive complaints, such as irritable bowel syndrome, constipation, indigestion, and associated conditions that can arise from eating inappropriate foods — for example, eczema, water retention, and circulation problems.

You should be treated only by an Ayurvedic physician with a full degree from a recognized university. Make sure that you do not accept treatment from any self-styled Ayurvedic practitioners since inappropriate treatment could cause damage to both your body and your mind.

How many sessions?

You may wish to visit your practitioner regularly in order to maintain good health. Much Ayurvedic medicine is preventive, but illnesses and diseases are also treated. The number of sessions needed to treat specific problems will depend on several factors, such as your age, the nature of your dosha imbalance, its severity, and the length of time you have had it. A condition such as irritable bowel syndrome could improve in two to six visits, while sinusitis might take five to ten.

What to expect

Ayurvedic treatment is normally extremely pleasant and gentle. Your practitioner is likely to recommend exercise, a suitable diet, herbal medicines, an external and internal detoxification program, and perhaps other therapies, such as marma therapy, gem therapy, or ways to relax through meditation and yoga. You may be surprised by the breadth and variety of the Ayurvedic discipline.

Qualities of a Good Physician

An Ayurvedic practitioner should have integrity as well as medical experience, embodying the following qualities:

- Purity of body and mind;

- Wide breadth of knowledge and excellent medical education;

- Training in both the theory and practice of medicine, as well as wide clinical experience.

AN AYURVEDIC CONSULTATION

An initial consultation usually concentrates on the diagnosis of any problems, and can take up to an hour. First you will be asked detailed questions about your health and lifestyle and the health of your parents. These factors will be reflected in the state of your doshas. The question session usually takes up about a third of the consultation time. The physician will also look at your eyes, tongue, fingernails, and other signs.

Questions about you

Your practitioner will want to know how you were as a child and teenager in order to determine your prakruthi (balanced state). Information about your lifestyle, diet, job, social behavior, symptoms, and likes and dislikes also aid the diagnosis. In addition, you will be asked about your digestion, appetite, and bowel movements.

Your tongue is an indicator of your state of health

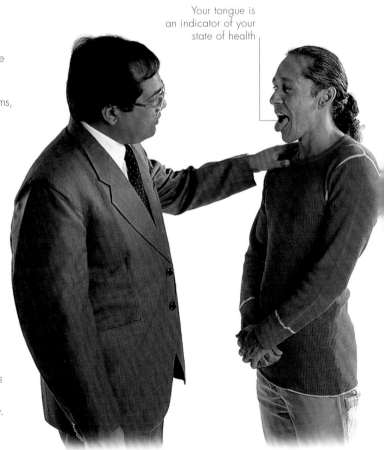

Experience & wisdom

Your Ayurvedic practitioner is drawing on the wisdom of a therapy that's helped hundreds of thousands of people, and prevented illness in even more.

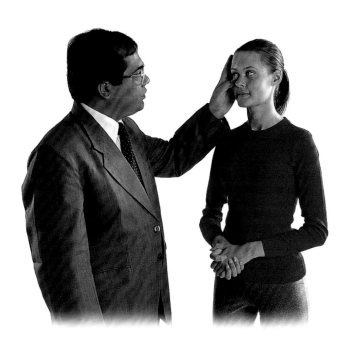

Changing your lifestyle

Your practitioner's aim will be to help you achieve long-lasting good health. You may have to make some lifestyle changes in order to achieve this and will have to stop whatever activity is causing disharmony, whether it is excessive drinking, overwork, or lack of sleep.

Eye to eye
The eyes are an obvious place to look for signs of imbalance or unhealthy activities.

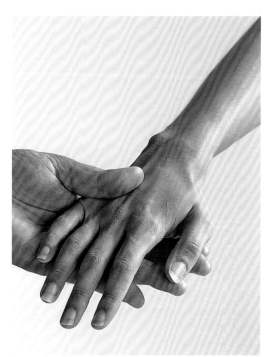

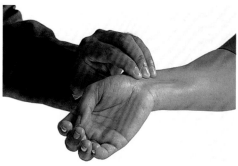

Pulse check
Different doshas have different pulses, and your pulse will be taken to help with diagnosis.

At your fingertips
The fingers and thumbs represent the five elements and provide clues about your health.

The Physical Examination

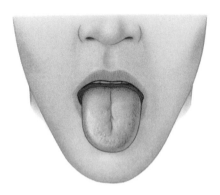

Reading the signs

Everything from your tongue to your fingernails will be assessed during an examination.

It normally takes about 30 minutes for an Ayurvedic practitioner to complete a physical examination, and you may be surprised by the level of care taken to investigate everything about you. Examinations may involve the ten-fold examination (see box) and/or the eight-fold examination. The eight-fold examination gives the practitioner an idea of the nature of any illness and your general condition. It will include an examination of your general appearance, tongue, skin, voice, pulse, eyes, urine, and stool.

Physical clues

Your tongue, for example, can provide a great deal of information about your dosha and your overall health. A kapha tongue has a white coating, a pitta tongue is yellow and red, while a vata tongue is very active. Your hands will also provide essential information about dosha imbalances, and your fingers and thumbs will tell your practitioner how each of the five elements in your body (and the organs to which they relate) are faring. Your thumbs relate to ether and the brain, your index fingers represent air and your lungs, your middle finger is fire and will provide clues to the health of your intestines, your ring finger relates to water (and therefore your kidneys), while your little finger represents earth and your heart.

Your practitioner will take your pulse. The pulse diagnosis is called *nadi shastra*, and your practitioner will feel (palpate) for three pulse points on the radial artery of each wrist. Each of the three pulse points relates to a dosha: the one on which the index finger rests is vata, the middle finger rests on pitta, and the ring finger feels for kapha. A dominant vata pulse is called the snake pulse because of its irregular sliding movement, a pitta pulse is called the frog, and the graceful pulse of kapha is the swan. These three points have up to 32 different qualities, which give essential information about your health: from the state of each organ and the quality of the blood, to the doshas that relate to the five elements.

Ten-fold Examination

This more detailed examination will assess your:

- Body constitution (*prakrithi*);
- Pathological state (*vikrithi*);
- Tissue vitality (*sara*);
- Body measurement (*pramana*);
- Physical build (*samhanana*);
- Adaptability (*satmya*);
- Psychic constitution (*sattva*);
- Digestive capacity (*ahara sakti*);
- Capacity for exercise (*vyayama sakti*);
- Age (*vaya*).

Medicines
Thousands of natural drugs are used in Ayurveda—guggul is used as an anti-inflammatory, however, it should not be used during pregnancy.

HOSPITAL TREATMENTS Some therapies, such as panchakarma,

involve consecutive treatments over several days and therefore require considerable commitment by the patient. They may be more easily given in a controlled environment, such as a hospital, so that the patient does not miss part of the treatments or combine them with other therapies.

A full range
Most Ayurvedic hospitals will offer a full range of Ayurvedic and yoga therapies as well as Ayurvedic herbs and medicines. The Ayurvedic Charitable Hospital in London, for example, stocks more than 2,000 medicines, powders, and oils. Only certified natural, herbal Ayurvedic formulations are used, and preparations are made on the day that the medicine is used.

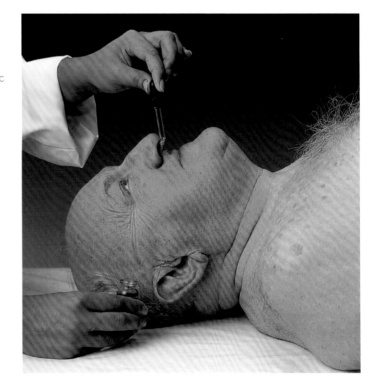

Nasya therapy
Medicated oils or powders are applied to the nostrils in nasya, often used for kapha-oriented disorders in the head area.

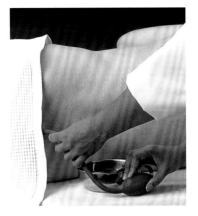

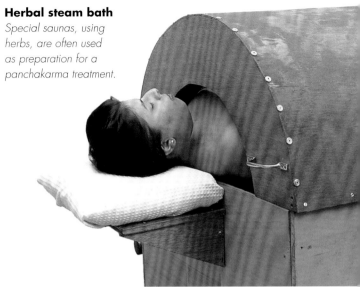

Herbal steam bath
Special saunas, using herbs, are often used as preparation for a panchakarma treatment.

Basti therapy
Herbal-oil enemas or douches are used to treat disorders caused by excess vata.

Complaints Treated in a Hospital

The following complaints may be effectively treated in a hospital environment:

- *Ama-vata/vata-rakta* (rheumatoid arthritis, gout, and other immune diseases);

- *Sandhi-vata* (osteoarthritis, degenerative arthritis);

- *Gradrasi-vata* (sciatica);

- *Avabaahuka* (painful shoulder syndrome, frozen shoulder);

- *Kati-graha/trika-graha* (lumbago, spondylitis);

- *Parkshaaghata* (hemiplegia, paraplegia);

- *Ardita* (facial paralysis);

- *Chittodwega/vishaada* (general anxiety disorders, depression);

- *Sthoulya* (obesity);

- *Madhumeha* (diabetes);

- *Shoolam/shirah shoolam* (chronic pain, headache, migraine);

- *Kampa-vata* (Parkinson's disease);

- *Tamaka-swasa* (bronchial asthma);

- *Amla-pitta* (acid-peptic diseases);

- *Mada/madaatyaya* (alcoholism, addiction);

- *Vibanda/anaaha/udaavarta* (constipation, flatulence, gas);

- *Atisaara* (chronic diarrhea);

- *Kustha* (skin diseases);

- *Yakrit-pleehodara* (liver disease, hepato-spleenomegaly);

- *Kridroga* (coronary artery disease).

An Ayurvedic Hospital

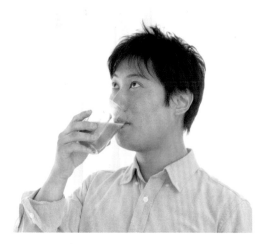

Cleansing the body
In virechana therapy, you take purgatives or laxatives to eliminate excess pitta.

those people whose conditions cannot benefit from Western medicine. It offers an opportunity for patients to receive full Ayurvedic treatment from highly trained Ayurvedic physicians, and patients are treated free of charge. Funding is by donation, which allows the facilities to be used by anyone, from any country, race, or religion around the world.

Besides receiving full residential care, patients at the hospital are put under careful supervision as dietary, lifestyle, and detoxification therapies are administered over consecutive days. Yoga therapy is also offered to patients.

Ayurvedic medicine enjoys popular support in India despite the growing use of Western medicine, and Western-trained doctors can be found working alongside Ayurvedic practitioners in many areas.

However, it was not until 2000 that the first Ayurvedic hospital in the West was opened in Britain. Founded by Gopi Warrier and based in London, the Ayurvedic Charitable Hospital aims to use the principles of ayurveda to cure

What is treated?

The hospital treats many chronic ailments, such as asthma, rheumatoid arthritis, colitis, cystitis, polymyalgia rheumatica (PMR), depression, and prostatitis. The treatments offered produce none of the side-effects that can be associated with drugs used in Western medicine.

The hospital does not, however, provide treatment for heart attacks, conditions requiring emergency surgery, or acute illnesses or infections.

Case History

Carol Johnson was 51 when she arrived at the hospital with progressive motor neurone disease. She was unable to stand, move her limbs, or even speak. Her muscle wasting was prominent and progressive, and she was clinically depressed. She had been treated by neurologists without experiencing much relief, and had been suffering the side-effects of the drugs she had been taking.

The physicians at the hospital found that she was a kapha-vata type, with an imbalance of vata. She was prescribed various treatments, notably nasya therapy, over 21 days. There were remarkable changes within three days, and these continued as therapy progressed. Her speech became clearer day by day, and the movement of her limbs improved as the weeks went by. As Carol noticed the improvements, she became more hopeful and her depression began to lift.

At the time of discharge, Carol could get up from her bed, stand without support, walk seven or eight steps without aid, and speak a few words clearly. She was no longer suffering from depression.

An Ayurvedic Degree

Most Ayurvedic physicians train in India, but there are now also degree programs in the U.K. and other countries—further evidence of the swing toward this ancient art of healing.

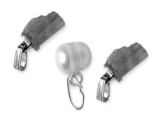

Natural energy

The natural energy of the earth is contained in gems, and these can affect your health.

AFTER TREATMENT

When a therapy session is over, looking after your mind and body should remain a priority, and your practitioner will give you advice on how to do this. In general, setting up a daily routine and practicing self-massage is a good start, but there are other ways in which you can pay attention to your spiritual and physical needs. Meditation, yoga, and good food should all be incorporated into your daily routine. You can also make changes to your energy levels by using gemstones.

Meditation

Without meditation (see pages 122–27), the true healing potential of Ayurvedic medicine cannot be realized. Mediation lets you settle into a state of profound stillness, which turns the mind inward to spirit and spiritual potential. It is rejuvenating and draws together the mind and the spirit.

Let thoughts come and go

Breathe deeply

Let your hands rest gently on your knees

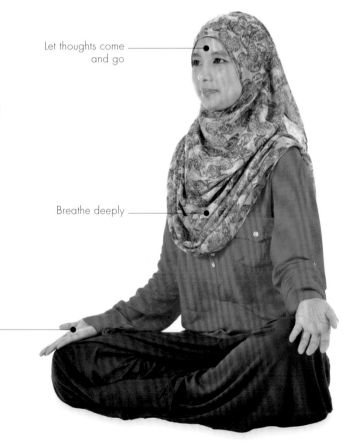

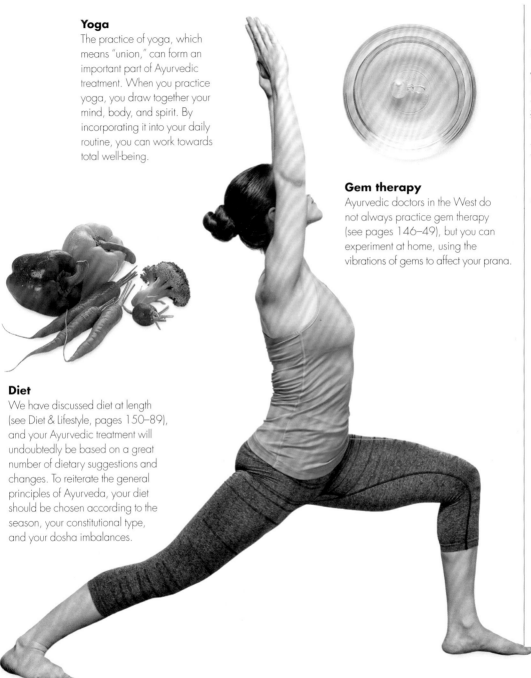

Yoga

The practice of yoga, which means "union," can form an important part of Ayurvedic treatment. When you practice yoga, you draw together your mind, body, and spirit. By incorporating it into your daily routine, you can work towards total well-being.

Gem therapy

Ayurvedic doctors in the West do not always practice gem therapy (see pages 146–49), but you can experiment at home, using the vibrations of gems to affect your prana.

Diet

We have discussed diet at length (see Diet & Lifestyle, pages 150–89), and your Ayurvedic treatment will undoubtedly be based on a great number of dietary suggestions and changes. To reiterate the general principles of Ayurveda, your diet should be chosen according to the season, your constitutional type, and your dosha imbalances.

Ayurvedic & Western Medicine

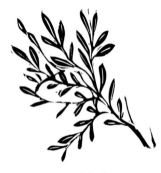

A natural balance

Ayurveda uses natural remedies and therapies to stimulate your body to heal itself.

It is important to understand the basic difference between Ayurveda and Western allopathic medicine. Western allopathic medicine currently tends to focus on symptomatology and disease, and primarily uses drugs and surgery to rid the body of pathogens or diseased tissue. Many lives have been saved by this approach. In fact, surgery is encompassed by Ayurveda. However, drugs, because of their toxicity, often weaken the body. Ayurveda does not focus on disease. Instead, Ayurveda maintains that all life must be supported by energy in balance. When there is minimal stress and the flow of energy within a person is balanced, the body's natural defenses will be strong and can more easily prevent disease.

Western medicine

Ayurveda is not a substitute for Western allopathic medicine. There are many instances when the disease process and acute conditions can best be treated with drugs or surgery. Ayurveda can be used in conjunction with Western medicine to make you less likely to be afflicted with disease, or to strengthen the body after drugs or surgery.

Ayurveda can also be effective in the treatment of conditions that Western medicine has not been able to address, such as asthma and eczema. In serious cases, conventional drugs may be used alongside Ayurvedic treatments at first, and then gently phased out.

Out of balance

Many illnesses are the cause of imbalance in some area of our life, and this is something that Western medicine often fails to address. By working to treat the root cause of disease, Ayurveda can be more successful than conventional medicine, and the results can be permanent, provided that you take steps to keep your lifestyle balanced after treatment.

Ayurveda comes into its own with many niggling health conditions that cannot be treated conventionally. Not sinister enough to be considered a disease, these symptoms are still uncomfortable. What we are often experiencing in these situations is imbalance, and that is precisely what Ayurveda treats so well.

Unique Insight

Ayurveda recognizes that each of us responds differently to the many aspects of life and possesses different strengths and weaknesses.

AYURVEDA AT HOME

To get the most from Ayurveda, you should see an Ayurvedic doctor, who can assess you and ascertain your constitutional type before prescribing treatment. However, there are plenty of ways to help yourself at home as well. Lots of the herbs and oils used can be found in your pantry. You can also choose a diet and exercises that best suit your lifestyle and your doshas.

Toxic build-up

There are some points to bear in mind when treating yourself at home. When using herbs, change them frequently to avoid a build-up of toxins and even a possible dependency or allergic reaction. Although these cases are rare, they can occur. Discontinue use immediately if you experience any discomfort.

An Ayurvedic doctor will give you a full assessment

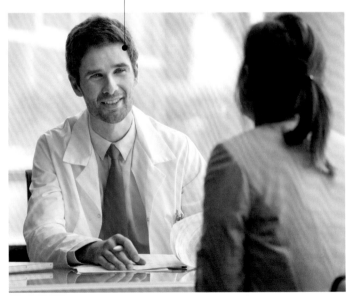

Ask for help

Before embarking on a self-help program, it's a good idea to get advice from a practitioner.

Home treatment

When used therapeutically, herbs can be very powerful and can have a profound effect on your body and constitution. Don't experiment with large quantities, and remember that "more" doesn't mean "more effective." Use small amounts to see if there is a noticeable effect.

Meditation

Open your mind with meditation, to experience healing and peace.

Self-massage

Use oils that are suitable for your dosha, and remember that they can be powerful tools.

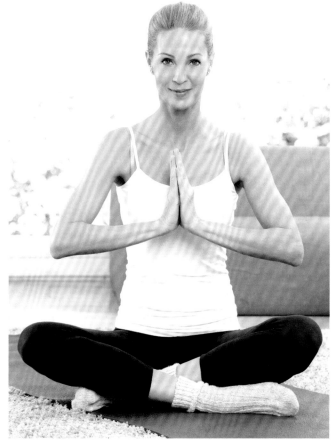

Before You Start

On the following pages there are some tried-and-tested remedies for common conditions. This is not to say that they are appropriate for you. Always get expert advice before starting an at-home medical program. It is important, no matter what your state of health, that you have your dosha assessed. If you get it wrong, you can cause great imbalance.

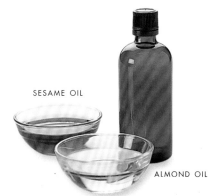

SESAME OIL

ALMOND OIL

Common Ailments

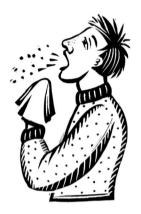

Not feeling well?

In Ayurveda, illness is caused by imbalance. Working out the cause will help you find a cure.

Many common ailments can be treated safely at home. Most treatments simply require thinking through the root cause of your condition and addressing that. Remember that, in Ayurvedic terms, the majority of ailments are simply symptoms of imbalance. By righting that imbalance, you will feel much better.

You will always need to work out your dosha type, and to follow the lifestyle suggestions for that type, in order to overcome illness. Herbs, crystals,

and oils can be used at home in small quantities to relieve symptoms (see box opposite for some useful herbs). If you see no change in your condition, see a practitioner.

Insomnia

Use nutmeg, valerian, and poppy, steeped in milk. Avoid vata-producing influences, such as stress, travel, erratic lifestyle, stimulants, and overwork. In the pitta dosha, insomnia is brought on by anger, jealousy, frustration, fever, or excess heat. Follow the lifestyle suggestions for pitta types (see pages 212–13 for summary), and massage brahmi oil into your head and feet.

Colds

Use herbs to decongest, balance, boost immunity, and warm. The most suitable are ginger, cinnamon, licorice, echinacea, angelica, dandelion, and fresh peppermint. Vata colds involve dry symptoms—ginger, cumin, and pippali are good for these. Pitta colds are heating, and there may be fever—use peppermint and sandalwood.

Kapha colds tend to be thick and heavy. Drink spiced teas of hot lemon, ginger, cinnamon, cloves, and tulsi, and add a little honey. Other useful herbs are pippali and peppermint. Saunas and hot baths could help to increase heat.

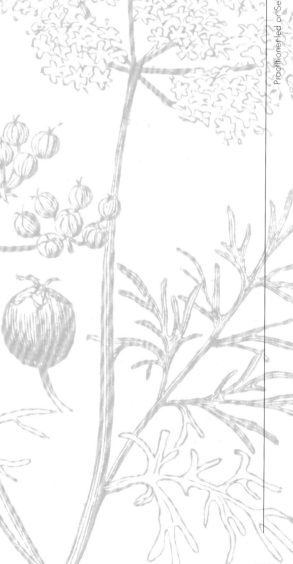

Herbs	Aliments
CILANTRO	Sinus problems, headaches, colds, and cystitis
MUSTARD OIL AND SEEDS	Headaches, fever, cold feet and hands, and rheumatism
CURRY LEAVES	Menstrual pain
GARLIC	Toothache, bacterial and fungal infections, viruses, candida, and diarrhea
GINGER	Indigestion, coughs and sore throats, and fungal infections
MUSTARD	Menstrual problems, diarrhea, fevers, indigestion, and hemorrhoids
GOTU KOLA	Balancing all three doshas and stimulating the circulatory system, strengthening memory, and improving concentration

What is your dosha?
Before embarking on any Ayurvedic program, you must be certain that you have your dosha type right.

AN AYURVEDIC LIFESTYLE
Whatever the state of your health, and whatever complaints you may be suffering from, you will undoubtedly benefit from living according to your dosha type. Throughout this book we have discussed dietary and lifestyle changes that can and should be made. The following lists give some quick tips on balancing your dosha type. If you can, practice these tips daily.

Vata
This dosha gives us the energy of movement. Adopting the following advice can prevent imbalance.
- Keep warm and avoid extreme cold.
- Stay calm.
- Have a regular routine.
- Get plenty of rest and try to go to bed at the same time every night.
- Eat warm foods and spices.
- Avoid eating cold, frozen, or raw foods.

Keeping warm
All doshas should dress warmly in winter, but this is particularly important for vata types.

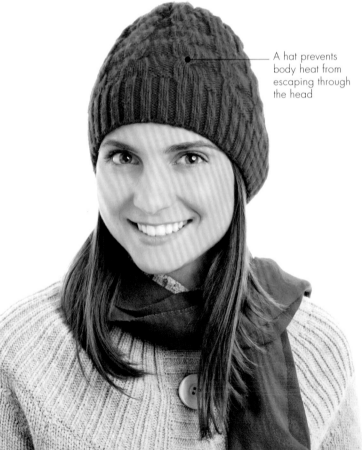

A hat prevents body heat from escaping through the head

Pitta

The following are ways to balance pitta, which provides the energy of digestion.

- Avoid excessive heat and excessive steam.
- Do not exercise when the weather is hot.
- Eat cooling foods.
- Avoid excessive oil.
- Limit salt intake.

Kapha

This dosha governs lubrication in the body. The following lifestyle changes are helpful.

- Keep active and take plenty of exercise.
- Don't sleep during the day.
- Vary your routine.
- Exclude heavy, fatty, and oily foods in your diet.
- Avoid dairy products.

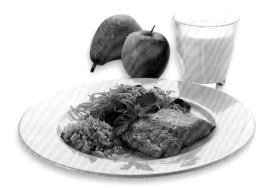

Dosha diet

The diet you adopt is crucial in Ayurveda; pitta types should eat plenty of cooling foods.

Finding a Balance

It is often difficult to make lifestyle changes, but any changes you make toward balancing your dosha will enhance your well-being. Don't be alarmed by the number of guidelines for Ayurvedic living. Most of them can be easily incorporated into daily life, and as your health improves, you'll find that you naturally choose a way of life that maintains that healthy balance.

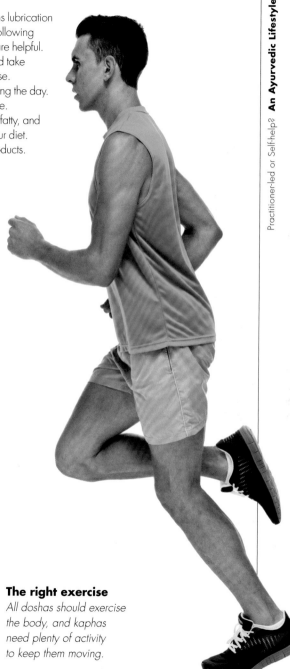

The right exercise

All doshas should exercise the body, and kaphas need plenty of activity to keep them moving.

Summary of the Doshas

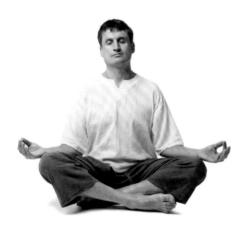

Inner being
*Knowing and respecting your
dosha will help you to reach a
natural state of well-being.*

Here, the three dosha types are summarized to help you to remember the key messages for each one. Keep the main points in mind on a daily basis.

Vata

Vata provides the essential motion for all bodily processes. It is most prominent in the fall and at the change of seasons. Routine is useful in assisting the vata individual effectively to ground all this moving energy. Since the attributes of vata are dry, light, cold, rough, subtle, mobile, and clear, any of these qualities in excess can cause imbalance. Frequent travel, especially by plane, loud noises, continual stimulation, drugs, sugar, and alcohol, all accentuate vata. Vata types have a hard time becoming and staying grounded. It is best for vatas to go to bed by 10 pm as they need more rest than the other types. In general, people with excessive vata respond most rapidly to warm, moist, slightly oily, heavy foods. Steam baths, humidifiers, and moisture in general are helpful. A daily oil massage before a bath or shower is recommended.

Pitta

Pitta types have many of the qualities of fire, which is hot, penetrating, sharp, and agitating. Similarly, pitta people have warm bodies, penetrating ideas, and sharp intelligence. When out of balance, they can become agitated and short-tempered. Since the attributes of pitta are oily, hot, light, mobile, dispersing, and liquid, an excess of any of these qualities aggravates pitta. Summer, the season of heat, is the pitta season, and many pitta disorders arise then. Diet and lifestyle changes focus on coolness. People with excessive pitta should not exercise in the heat.

Kapha

Kapha types have strength, endurance, and stamina. In balance, they tend to have sweet, loving dispositions. Kapha types are attracted to sweet, salty, and oily foods, but their constitutions are balanced by astringent, pungent, and bitter tastes. Kapha people can become more irritated as the moon gets full, because there is a tendency for water retention at that time. Winter is the time when kapha accumulates, and following the kapha-balancing changes is important during that season.

Check Your Dosha

Before embarking on any Ayurvedic program, you must make sure that your dosha has been properly assessed.

213

LIVING A HAPPY LIFE

The ultimate aim of all of us is to have a long and happy life. Ayurveda can work on your mind, body, and spirit to help you achieve just that. The aim of Ayurveda is more than adding years to your life—it aims to add life to your years. Only when body, mind, and soul live in harmony is complete health possible. Ayurveda addresses all of these elements with a broad-ranging, detailed series of treatments that form your lifestyle for today and for the future.

Stress

Stress is very much a modern complaint, yet the treatise of Ayurveda outlines very clearly the damage done by stressful living. Ayurveda teaches right living, and that means living well, happily, and for the good of yourself and others. If you are running the rat race every day, working too hard, in an unhappy relationship, obsessed by success and money, or if you never see your family and never have time to relax, it is fairly obvious that you are not living in the right way. Ayurveda offers you a chance to change your life and yourself.

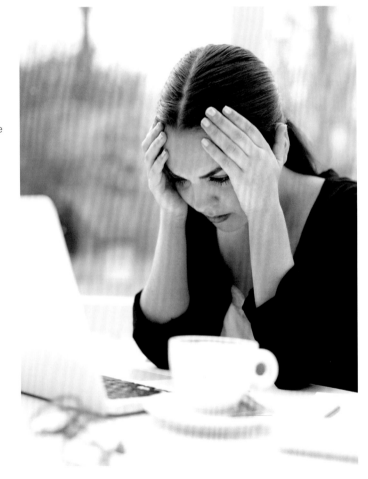

Look at your life

If stress features strongly in your life, your health and happiness will suffer, and your body will be thrown out of balance.

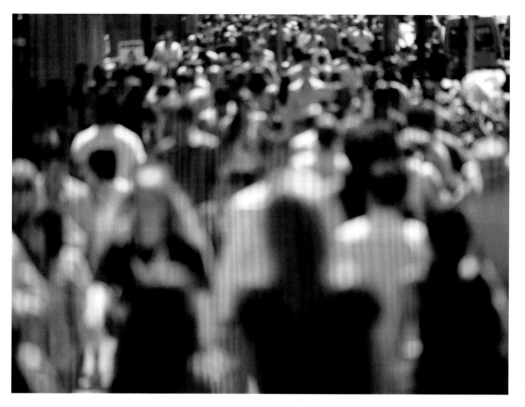

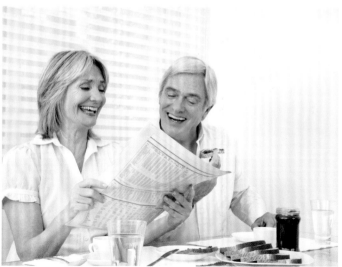

Escaping the rat race

Taking time for yourself can help to balance the stresses caused by the Western lifestyle.

Aging

In Ayurvedic theory, the idea of aging is called an "intellectual error," as people are regarded only in terms of their physical condition. Forget your chronological age. Focus instead on the capability and freshness of your mind, and allow yourself to become ageless.

GLOSSARY

Agni the term for all fires, from digestion to the essence of cosmic fire.

Ama a general term for the toxins that are produced by improper metabolic functioning.

Chakras seven centers of energy in the body.

Charaka Samhita one of the first substantial texts on Ayurveda, compiled about 3,000 years ago.

Dhaatus the body tissues, which are plasma, blood, muscle, fat, bone, marrow and nerves, and the reproductive tissues.

Dosha invisible force (the word actually means "fault" or "mistake"). There are three doshas (vata, pitta, and kapha) which are responsible for all biological and psychological functioning of the mind and body.

Ghee clarified butter.

Jyotish Indian astrology, used in Ayurvedic medicine to aid with healing.

Kapha one of the three doshas, comprising water and earth elements.

Malas the waste products— sweat, urine, and feces.

Marma points these are points on the body significant to the flow of life energy.

Ojas a hormone-like substance which integrates body, mind, and spirit. Ojas transmits energy from mind to body and controls immunity.

Panchakarma a five-stage purification program.

Panchamahabhutas the five great elements or states of material existence, which are ether (space), air, fire, water, and earth.

Purvakarma Cleansing program, which is used to prepare the body for panchakarma therapies.

Pitta one of the three doshas, comprising fire and water elements.

Prakrithi first action—our inherent nature or constitution.

Prana life force.

Rajasic the average state of mind in which mood swings are common, as well as overindulgence.

Rasa tastes, and the emotions derived from them.

Rasayana rejuvenation therapy, to return your body, mind, and spirit to an earlier state of integration.

Sattvic the highest state of mind, characterized by equilibrium. Attained through spiritual development.

Tamasic the lowest state of mind, characterized by negativity, selfishness, lack of energy, and poor diet.

Vata one of the three doshas, which comprises air and space.

Vedas India's ancient books of wisdom.

Vikruthi the changeable and current state of your health, which is a temporary condition expressed as the state of the three doshas.

FURTHER READING

Bhishagratna, K.L. (translator) *Sushruta Samhita.* Chaukhambha, India, 1981.

Chopra, Deepak. *Ageless Body, Timeless Mind: A Practical Alternative to Growing Old.* Rider Books, U.K., 1993.

Chopra, Deepak. *Perfect Health: The Complete Mind/Body Guide.* Bantam Books, London, 1990.

Chopra, Deepak. *Quantum Healing: Exploring the Frontiers of Mind/Body Medicine.* Bantam Books, U.S., 1991.

Dash, Bhagwan. *Basic Principles of Ayurveda.* Concept Publishing, India, 1980.

Dash, Vaidya Bhagwan and Acarya Manfred M. Junius. *A Handbook of Ayurveda.* Concept Publishing, India, 1983.

Gerson, Scott. *Ayurveda: The Ancient Healing Art.* Element, U.K., 1993.

Godagama, Dr. Shantha. *The Handbook of Ayurveda.* Kyle Cathie, London, 1997.

Lad, Vasant. *The Complete Book of Ayurvedic Home Remedies.* Piatkus, London, 1998.

Lad, Vasant, and Dr. David Frawley. *The Yoga of Herbs: An Ayurvedic Guide to Herbal Medicine.* Lotus Press, U.S., 1988.

Murthy, Prof. K.R. Srikanta. *Madhava Nidanam (Roga Viniscaya) of Madhavakara: A Treatise on Ayurveda.* Chaukhambha Orietanlia, India, 1987.

Sharma, Pandit Shiv. *Ayurvedic Medicine, Past and Present.* Dabur Publications, India, 1975.

Sharma, P.V. *Caraka Samhita.* Chaukhambha Orietanlia, Inida, U.K., 1981.

Svoboda, Dr. Robert. *Prakruti: Your Ayurvedic Constutition.* Geocom, U.S., 1989.

Warrier, Gopi, and M.D. Deepika Gunawant *The Complete Illustrated Guide to Ayurveda: The Ancient Healing Tradition.* Element Books, U.K., 1997.

Wilson, H.H. *The Vishnu Purana, a System of Hindu Mythology and Tradition.* Panthi Pustak, India, 1961.

The Bhagavad Gita—any edition.

Translation by Board of Scholars. *The Siva-purana.* Motilal Banarsidass, India, 1970.

USEFUL ADDRESSES

USA

The Ayurvedic Institute

www.ayurveda.com
Established in 1984, The Ayurvedic Institute is one of the leading Ayurvedic schools and health spas outside of India.

National Ayurvedic Medicine Association (NAMA)

www.ayurvedanama.org
A national organization aiming to preserve, protect, and promote the practice of Ayurveda and to provide leadership within the profession.

American Institute of Vedic Studies

www.vedanet.com
An online educational resource providing publications on Ayurveda, Yoga-Vedanta, Vedic astrology, and their interconnections.

California College of Ayurveda

www.ayurvedacollege.com
Founded in 1995, the California College of Ayurveda was the first school, outside of India, to gain government approval and provide formal education in Ayurvedic Medicine.

American Botanical Council

www.abc.herbalgram.org/site/PageServer
An organization offering advice and information on the safe and effective use of plants and medicinal herbs.

Napralert (Natural Product Database)

www.napralert.org
A comprehensive database of natural products; including over 200,000 scientific papers and reviews.

UK

College of Ayurveda

www.ayurvedacollege.co.uk
An Ayurvedic college offering hands-on practical knowledge and skills by trained practitioners through a series of seminars and workshops.

The British Association of Accredited Ayurvedic Practitioners (BAAP)

www.britayurpractitioners.com
A professional affiliate of the British Ayurvedic Medical Council, the BAAP was established to help promote Ayurveda in the West.

Yoga Biomedical Trust

www.yogatherapy.org
A charity whose aim is to facilitate the development of yoga as a holistic therapy for the treatment of medical conditions.

Maharishi Ayurveda

www.maharishi.co.uk
A website offering high quality, authentic Ayurvedic products, health guides, recipes, and videos.

Neal's Yard Remedies

www.nealsyardremedies.com
Originating in Covent Garden, London, Neal's Yard Remedies is a company aiming to bring the expertise of apothecary, and a holistic approach, to their health and beauty products.

CANADA

Canadian Ayurveda Members Alliance

www.camayurveda.com
A national organization that represents the Ayurvedic profession in Canada, and whose mission is to preserve, protect, and promote the practice.

WEBSITE ADDRESSES

The following websites give general information about Ayurveda:
www.ayurveda.com
www.worldwidehealthcenter.net

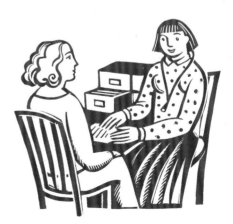

INDEX

a

aftercare 202–3
aging 105, 138–39, 215
agni *see* metabolism
air element 34, 54–55
aloe vera 98
ama 25, 65, 102, 172, 188–89
appearance 30–31, 35, 39, 43, 48–49
appetite 174–75
arms, marma points 86–87
Asparagus racemosus 103,143
astringent foods 160–63
astrology 142–47
Ayurvedic Charitable Hospital 198, 200

b

back, marma points 86
balance
  concept of 24–25
  for the doshas 36–37, 40–41, 44–45, 178
basti therapy 72, 199
bhastika breath 121
bitter foods 160–63
black pepper 99
blood 60, 72–73
body
  and the doshas 58–59
  misuse 28
  tissues 60–62
  waste 64–65
  weight 176–78
bone 60, 88
breathing exercises 109, 118–21

c

caraway 99
carrier substances 94
chakras 90–93, 149
chandrashtama 145
Charaka Samhita 14, 15, 21, 25, 102
childhood 139
Chinese medicine 16, 88–89
chronobiology 132–33
cinnamon 99
cobra position 115
colds 208–9
color visualization 93
common aliments 208–9
consultations 192–95
creams 100

d

daily living 140–41
dairy foods 154, 157
daytime 133–35, 140–41
demonic possession 15
detoxification 24–25, 68, 70–75, 180–81, 186–89
dhaatus 60–61
diagnosis 46
diet 69, 150–89, 203
  and detoxification 75, 180–81, 186–89
  doshas and 47, 158–72, 174–78, 184–85
  fasting 180–81
  food categories 154–55, 164–65
  foods as medicine 182–83
  guidelines 156–57
  and life energy 63
  and metabolism 172–73
  seasonal 137, 162–63
  six tastes 158–61
disease
  causes of 20, 28–29, 56–57, 62, 65
  common 208–9
doshas 29–51
  see also kapha; pitta; vata
  and aging 138–39
  assessment of 46–51
  Ayurvedic time clock 133–35
  balanced 36–37, 40–41, 44–45, 178
  and the body 58–59
  and breathing 119
  and colds 208–9
  and detoxification 72, 74
  and diet 158–72, 174–78, 184–85
  herbs for 97
  imbalanced 35–37, 40–41, 44–45, 56–61
  and insomnia 208
  and lifestyle 210–11
  physical exercise for 106–7, 115
  and seasonal cycles 136–37
  and the senses 130, 131
  summary of 212–13
douches 101
drinks 63, 147, 155

e

earth element 42, 54–55
eight branches 18–19
elements 34, 38, 42, 54–55, 131, 160–61

energy
  kundalini 90, 92
  ojas 62–63
  prana 88, 118
ether element 34, 54–55
eye examinations 195

f

fall 163
fasting 180–81
fat 60
fecal waste 64–65
fingers 195, 196
fire element 38, 54–55
fish 155
fish asana 116
foot massage 83, 85
fruit 155, 157

g

garlic 182, 209
gem therapy 146–49, 203
ginger 182, 209
Greek medicine 16

h

happiness 214–15
head, marma points 86–87
healing, types of 128
health 24–27, 152–53
herbal teas 180, 181
herbalism 68–69, 94–101
  for common ailments 208–9
  herbal properties 96–97
  regenerative 103
  self-help 206–7
  steam baths 75, 199
  toxic build-up 206

using herbs 100–101
weight control 177
history of Ayurveda 9, 14–17
holism 18
hospital treatment 198–201

i

imbalance 205
  and appetite 175
  and body weight 176, 178
  concept of 24–25, 28–31
  in the dhaatus 60–61
  in the doshas 35–37, 40–41,
    44–45, 56–61
  seven stages 56–57
infusions 100
insomnia 208

k

kapha 42–45
  and appetite 174
  assessment of 49, 50
  balanced 44–45
  and the body 59
  and body weight 177
  breathing exercises for 119
  characteristics 31–33, 35,
    42–43, 213
  and colds 208–9
  and diet 47, 158–59, 162,
    170–72, 184–85
  gem therapy 149
  herbs for 97, 103
  imbalanced 44–45
  and lifestyle 211
  marma therapy 86–87
  massage oils for 81

physical exercise for
  106–7, 115
pulse checks for 197
rhythm of life 139
seasonal cycles 136
and the senses 131
time cycles 133, 135
types of 45
karma 20–23
kundalini energy 90, 92

l

legs, marma points 86–87
life, rhythm of 138–39
lifestyle 150–89, 195,
  210–11
long pepper 103
longevity 27, 43
Lord Brahma 9, 15
lunar stars 143, 144–45

m

malas 64–65
manasa prakrithi 53
mantras 126, 128–29
marma therapy 68, 86–89,
  92
marrow 60
massage 68, 70–71,
  76–85, 186, 207
meditation 122–29, 202,
  207
metabolism 61, 172–73
middle age 139
mind
  assessment 50–51
  and body weight 179
  constitution 52–53

moon 143–45
moral principles 153
motor neurone disease 201
muscle 60, 88

n
nasya therapy 73, 198
nature 132–33
neck, marma points 86–87
nerves 60
nighttime 133, 135, 141

o
oils 68, 70–71, 74–77, 79–81,
   101, 207
ojas 62–63
old age 139
onion 183

p
panchakarma 25, 68, 72–75
physical examinations 196–97
physical exercise 105, 106–17,
   187, 211
pitta 38–41
   and appetite 174
   assessment of 49, 50
   and the body 58, 59
   breathing exercises 119
   characteristics 31–33, 38–39,
      212–13
   and colds 208
   and detoxification 72
   and diet 47, 158–59, 163,
      168–69, 184–85
   fasting 181
   gem therapy 148
   herbs for 97, 103

imbalanced 40–41
   and insomnia 208
   and lifestyle 211
   marma therapy 86–87
   massage oils for 80
   physical exercise for 106–7,
      115
   pulse checks for 197
   rhythm of life 139
   seasonal cycles 136–37
   and the senses 131
   time cycles 133, 135
   types of 39
plough asana 116, 117
positive thought/action 104,
   152–53
practitioners 190–201
   consultations 192–95
   and diet 185
   hospital treatments 198–201
   physical examinations
      196–97
   qualifications 201
   qualities 193
   and self-help 206
prakruthi state 30
prana 68, 81, 88, 118
pranayama 109, 118–21
pulse checks 195, 196–97
pungent foods 160–62
purgation therapy 72, 199
purvakarma 68, 70–71,
   74–75

r
rajasic food 164–65
rajasic healing 128
rajasic mind 52, 53

raktamokshana 72–73
rasayana 69, 102–5
reincarnation 20
rejuvenation therapy 69,
   102–5
relaxation techniques 109, 117,
   122–29
routines, daily/ seasonal 69

s
salty foods 160–61, 163
salute to the sun asana 110–11
samana see herbalism
sattvic foods 164, 189
sattvic healing 128
sattvic mind 52–53
seasons
   cycles 29, 132–33, 136–37,
      187
   food and 162–63, 184
self-help 27, 202–3, 206–11
   detoxification 188–89
   herbalism 206–9
   and lifestyle 210–11
   massage 80–85, 207
   meditation 207
senses
   stimulation 28
   training 130–31
sex 153
Shiva 15
shodana see detoxification
shoulder stands 117
snehana see massage
sour foods 158, 160–61, 163
space element 34, 54–55
spiritual healing 69, 152–53
spring 162, 187

squats 113
steam baths 75, 199
stress 36, 125, 214–15
stretches 112–13
summer 163
suppositories 101
sweat therapy (swedana) 65, 70, 80
sweet foods 158, 160–61, 163

t
tablets 100
tamasic food 165
tamasic healing 128
tamasic mind 52, 53
tastes, six 158–61
theja 62
theory 26
time 29, 132–35
tinctures 100
tongues 196
toxic build-up 206
treatments 66–149
tree asana 114
tridoshas see doshas
trunk, marma points 87
turmeric 182, 183
twists 113

u
urinary system 64

v
vamana 73
vata 34–37
  and appetite 174
  assessment of 48, 50
  balanced 36–37
  and the body 58, 59
  and body weight 176–77
  breathing exercises for 119
  characteristics 30, 32–35, 212
  and colds 208
  and diet 47, 158–59, 163, 166–67, 184
  fasting 181
  gem therapy 147–48
  herbs for 97, 103
  imbalanced 35–37
  and lifestyle 210
  marma therapy 86–87
  massage oils for 80
  and metabolism 172
  physical exercise for 106–7, 115
  pulse checks for 197
  rhythm of life 139
  seasonal cycles 136
  and the senses 130
  time cycles 133–34
  types of 33
Vedas 9, 15, 16
vikruthi state 31
virechana 72
vitality breath 120
vomiting, therapeutic 73

w
water element 38, 42, 54–55
weight 176–78
Western medicine 12, 17, 204–5
winter 163, 187
winter cherry 103

y
yoga 27, 108–21, 203
  breathing 118–21
  exercises 108–17

ACKNOWLEDGMENTS

The publisher would like to thank the following for the kind loan of props for the photography:
Cargo HomeShop, London; The Ayurvedic Trading Company; Mysteries, London;
Neal's Yard Remedies, London; and Debbie Moore for Pineapple, London.

Special thanks go to The Ayurvedic Charitable Hospital, London, and Dr. Dattani,
Dr. Malagi, Dr. Indulal, and Dr. Gunawant for help with this book and the case history.
Thanks also to Mark Ansari, Denise Christian, Michaela Clarke, Ben Evans, Jamie Hickton,
Miranda La-Crette, and Louise Sweeney for their help with the photography.

PICTURE ACKNOWLEDGMENTS

Every effort has been made to trace copyright holders and obtain permission. The publishers apologize
for any omissions and would be pleased to make any necessary changes at subsequent printings

Alamy/ imageBROKER: 22b; mediacolor's: 73. **Bridgeman Art Library/** India, Office Library,
London: 15t. **Getty/** Bettmann / Contributor: 17, 134t; Paul Beinssen: 15b; Herve BRUHAT / Contributor:
74t; Dinodia Photo: 11; Fancy/Veer/Corbis: 46b; Michael Fellner: 9; Frederic Soltan: 129; PhotoAlto/Eric
Audras: 206; Vaidya Dhanvantari, Supreme Saint of Ayurveda Medicine, India School/Private Collection/
Dinodia: 14b; Matthew Wakem: 67, 205. **iStock/** 4x6: 107l, 175, 211r; andresr: 157t; Silvia Boratti:
55l; byheaven: 95t; Christopher Futcher: 139t; Mendelex_photography: 210b; Sonya_illustration: 91; Mark
Strozier: 53; thesomegirl: 151. **Shutterstock/** Africa Studio: 155c, 159b, 168r; azure1: 158; Yana
Alisovna: 30, 34, 38b, 42b, 46t, 51, 54b, 55r, 58t, 59, 130r, 135t, 166t, 168t, 170t, 210t;
Alohaflaminggo: 122t; artpixelgraphy Studio: 202b; Bandido Images: 95b; binik: 130–131; BLACKDAY:
33; Blinka: 141; blvdone: 215t; Natalie Board: 170r; Rommel Canlas: 174; Andy Dean Photography:
138; deeepblue: 153; Dragon Images: 178; Elena Elisseeva: 155b; Elovich: 182b; Evikka: 158; Ewais:
155t; f9photos: 90t, 203tl; fizkes: 63l, 106b; Flashon Studio: 106t; gary yim: 123bl; George Rudy: 179t;
Daniel Gilbey Photography - My portfolio: 101; GlebStock: 193; Joe Gough: 179b; Antonio Guillem: 107t;
JIANG HONGYAN: 182c; Image Point Fr: 85; Jasmina007: 121; Julenochek: 212; Kinga: 207t; Robert
Kneschke: 215b; Konstanttin: 165; kosmofish: 123t; kurhan: 139b, 187l; Lightspring: 54t; lightwavemedia:
197; lipik: 102b; Nina Lishchuk: 2; Little_Desire: 61; Dmitri Ma: 65; Mariyana M: 162t;
mimagephotography: 23, 125; Monkey Business Images: 105; morgenstjerne: 149; M. Unal Ozman: 158;
Nagib: 123br; Kritsada Namborisut: 166b; Nila Newsom: 13; Ilyashenko Oleksiy: 14t; ostill: 128; Pan
Stock: 183r; paulista: 154t; David Pereiras: 177; Photographee.eu: 72, 182t; photomak: 26; Pikoso.kz:
27, 109, 113; Piotr Krzeslak: 133, 57, 74b; pixelparticle: 142b; polkadot_photo: 200; Poznyakov: 77;
redstone: 158; Elena Schweitzer: 63cr; Serg64: 213; sergo iv: 29; Elena Shashkina: 173; sheff: 103r;
shooarts: 93; Smart-foto: 143t; Olaf Speier: 69; Marco Speranza: 62t; Vladyslav Starozhylov: 161;
stockcreations: 185; STUDIO GRAND OUEST: 191; subarashii21: 86, 87; Syda Productions: 122b;
Timolina: 122b, 159c; Aleksandar Todorovic: 186b; Anatoly Tiplyashin: 63tr; Victor Tongdee: 51;
Elena Trukhina: 63cr; Tspider: 25; Uber Images: 214; Vadven: 137; vaivirga: 98; Valentyn Volkov: 186t;
viki2win: 21; Viktor1: 158; Chursina Viktoriia: 63tr; v.s.anandhakrishna: 22t; Lilyana Vynogradova: 63cr;
Filip Warulik: 168l; Steven Wright: 145; MAHATHIR MOHD YASIN: 158.